PREVENTING DECL|NE

ADVANCES IN THE MEDICAL TREATMENT OF
HEARING LOSS & TINNITUS

DR. KEITH N. DARROW, PH.D., CCC-A
NEUROSCIENTIST, AUDIOLOGIST & CERTIFIED DEMENTIA PRACTITIONER

Preventing Decline: Advances in the Medical Treatment of Hearing Loss & Tinnitus
Dr. Keith N. Darrow

Disclaimer: The materials presented in this handbook are not meant to substitute for sound medical advice. While the author and the publisher have exercised their best efforts in preparing this handbook, they make no representations or warranties with respect to the accuracy or completeness of the content of this book and specifically disclaim any implied warranties of results or accuracy for a particular purpose. No warranty may be created or extended by sales representatives or written sales materials.

The advice and strategies contained herein may not be suitable for your situation and are provided to supplement your common sense, not substitute for it. You should consult with a professional where appropriate. Neither the publisher nor author shall be liable for any loss of profit or any other commercial damages, included but not limited to special, incidental, consequential, or other damages.

ISBN: 979-8-4869-9084-7

From my family to yours.

Thanks for all love and support of my family
(Laura, EMC[D,] my mother and many others) and my partners.
Because of you, this mission is possible . . . and achievable!

CONTENTS

HOW CAN I WRITE A REVIEW IN A FEW WORDS, WHEN I COULD write a book about how my life has changed since finding Dr. Darrow. His book *Stop Living in Isolation* described my life perfectly. It is going on three years since my first appointment when I walked in feeling apprehensive, but the best thing is that now I can understand the person who I always thought was mumbling, and the other one who always spoke in whispers, or too fast. Our big family gatherings are once again joyful now that I can follow and join in several conversations going on at once. I could go on and on. I am eternally grateful to Dr. Darrow and his wonderful staff for giving me my life back. You just can't put a price on that.

Jane H.
Patient at Hearing & Brain Center, Massachusetts
Excellence In Audiology Member

FOREWORD

WHY YOU NEED TO READ THIS BORING LITTLE BOOK!

My name is Dr. Keith N. Darrow, and I hold a Ph.D. in Speech and Hearing Bioscience from a joint Harvard Medical School and M.I.T. program. The reason I decided to become a Neuroscientist, a Clinical Audiologist and Certified Dementia Practitioner—instead of joining the ski patrol or becoming a handsome actor on Broadway—can be found in the pages at the end of this book.

Because this book is about you, or your spouse, or your parent and not about me. It's about the information you need to know to make intelligent, responsible decisions about your loved one's hearing health, brain health, self-esteem and social interactions...of a permanent, lifelong nature. It's about helping you understand what you can do every day to live more confidently, remain independent and how you can prevent dementia. This book is about providing education.

Perhaps you are one of the too many adults in our society who are beginning to decline and are living with untreated hearing loss and think *'ah, it's not a big deal that I can't hear great because this is normal as we get older'*. Or, maybe your loved ones invested in clunky old hearing aids and still walk around saying 'HUH?'or 'What?' all the time. I wrote this book to help you and your family make intelligent, informed, and responsible decisions about your health, to help you understand treatment options when it comes to hearing loss and tinnitus, and to help you decide how **you** want to age.

Throughout this book, I will address some of the most common questions my patients ask, and I will walk you through some of the common struggles I see families suffer through. As I tell all of my patients, *your ability to stay part of the conversation and remain independent impacts everybody around you!* I want you (and everyone of my patients) to understand the answers to these questions: Can I really prevent cognitive decline and dementia? Does he/she really NEED to treat mild hearing loss or tinnitus? Why do I need to treat my hearing loss and tinnitus? And If I chose to do so, **when** should I do it?? Who should I trust to provide me with the best treatment? How will we know if we can afford it and that we're not being ripped off? What do I do if I believe a loved one is starting to decline?

This book isn't *Fifty Shades of Gray*. I just can't make it that exciting. But if you will take the time to read this book, you will KNOW nearly everything you need to know to confidently make decisions about you or your loves one's hearing or tinnitus treatment and future livelihood.

Remember this: ***Aging is inevitable; but decline is optional!***

My first message is simple: It's not 1982. Not only has everything changed in our society—we live longer and more active lives—but when it comes to treating hearing loss and tinnitus not all treatments are created equal. NOT EVEN CLOSE. Long gone are the days of thinking there was nothing we could do to prevent memory loss and dementia as we got older. Also, the days of horrible, unsightly big beige bananas that your parents or grandparents used to wear are bygone relics. No longer do you have to traipse across town to the 'hearing doctor' to have the squealing turned down or have the plastic tubing changed because it turned hard and yellow. And no longer will a patient ever say 'I have to take my hearing aids off when I go to restaurants (or church, or family gatherings)'.

The technology we use to treat hearing loss and tinnitus is but one aspect of the number of options to consider when treating hearing loss and tinnitus. You never want to equate your hearing and brain health to buying something off the shelf at a big-box store, a retail pharmacy or (heaven forbid) from the internet! I shutter to think that so many patients think the medical treatment of hearing loss boils down to 'hey, I need a widget to help me hear better—what's it gonna cost me?'.

With that said, I understand that my patients do wonder about the technology we use to treat hearing loss. Like Baskin Robbins, there are lots of 'flavors' available to choose from and it can be overwhelming. Today's technology can be invisible, worn in the ear or behind the ear, can be semi-implanted and worn for months at a time. Today's technology is also safer, fully automatic (which means *no more button!*), Bluetooth enabled and waterproof. Today's technology is built around you living an active lifestyle and not worrying about your hearing. New treatments can restore your hearing in noisy situations so that you never miss another part of the conversation.

When I was growing up my own grandmother didn't get the treatment she needed because traditional hearing aids didn't provide the benefit that her hearing and brain needed.

We watched as she aged and separated herself from the family and all of her friends. We sat by, helpless, as she became riddled with dementia and was nothing more than a body in the room. Nobody should have to go through what my grandmother went through ever again.

My second message is: ***This Is More Than Just Traditional Hearing Aids!***

When seeking treatment from a hearing healthcare provider—you are in for a real treat! You must understand that hearing healthcare is not a simple financial transaction wherein you purchase a traditional hearing aid and stick it in your ear. That is like thinking diabetes only needs attention when your foot needs to be amputated, or like getting your tires checked when the tow truck comes to pick you up from getting a flat and being stranded in the pouring rain. YIKES!

We must be proactive with our health. We must be involved in our healthcare decisions. And we must accept that hearing healthcare is necessary, requires commitment (from both the patient and the provider) and that you treat your hearing loss and tinnitus to prevent further damage that may result from untreated or *under*treated hearing loss...including increased risk of falls, dementia, and even premature death.

Treatment check-ups by an Excellence In Audiology Certified Specialist starting at age fifty is a proper part of healthy aging. In many cases, prevention is less troublesome and way less costly. Remember, as with most medical conditions like heart disease, diabetes, cancer, etc., it is important to *catch it early and treat it early!*

In summary, (and this is just in case you don't have the time or you are too busy to read the entire book) here is why it is important to seek medical treatment for your hearing loss and tinnitus:

1. People who can hear in noise stay more active, participate in more social and family activities, maintain their independence, and stay in their home longer.

2. People who treat their hearing loss can reduce their risk of cognitive decline, memory loss and dementia.

3. People who treat their hearing loss may reduce or eliminate their tinnitus.

4. People who can hear properly feel better about themselves and that can greatly increase their confidence and livelihood.

So, do not put it off. Do not wait another day. Hearing loss isn't something that you can 'grow out of' or 'manage on your own'. The problems that come with hearing loss only get worse and harder to treat the longer they go untreated (or under-treated).

PREVENTING DECLINE: ADVANCES IN THE MEDICAL TREATMENT OF HEARING LOSS AND TINNITUS

Memory loss, cognitive decline and dementia are **not** a normal part of aging. Struggling to hear in noise, groups, church or family activities is also not normal—and it certainly isn't easy to live with. As we age, losing our metal faculties, having more 'senior moments' and missing out on the conversations around us makes us, or our loved ones, become self-conscious—painfully self-conscious—and embarrassed and frustrated. No one should ever say "*No thanks, dear, I'd rather just stay home and watch television*" because they are worried they are getting 'too old'.

Loneliness has skyrocketed since the pandemic of 2020 forced millions of American seniors into social isolation. Inactive and unengaged seniors will be an epidemic of its own on our families and society, affecting everything from the knowledge base of our communities to a strain on our healthcare system and overwhelmed assisted living centers. But it doesn't stop there. Untreated, and under-treated hearing loss, will significantly increase the likelihood of dementia, Falling, Institutionalization, and pre-mature death of our loved ones.

Hearing loss is the third most common chronic condition affecting our seniors and when treated, is the single most modifiable risk factor for the prevention of dementia. This is a medical condition and is a serious detriment to overall health and well-being.

So, read this book. Be informed. Be able to ask smart questions. Be able to do the right thing. I guarantee you'll be much better able to correctly and confidently make good choices for your loved ones by simply reading this book.

PREVENTING DECLINE

I HAD MY FIRST HEARING ASSESSMENT AND COGNITIVE WORK up this week. I learned so much from Dr. Darrow and was so impressed by the extensive testing and research. I felt comfortable through my entire exam and appreciated all their knowledge about a subject (for which I clearly did not know enough about). I am referring my parents especially to get tested and am so happy I took the plunge and got evaluated. Fantastic group of professionals. Thank you!

Susan C.
Patient at Hearing & Brain Centers, Massachusetts
Excellence In Audiology Member

PREVENTING DECLINE

CHAPTER 1

WHY IS MY HEARING SO IMPORTANT?

If you are like many who are weighing the *'yes/no'* decision of hearing healthcare, or maybe in the *'do it now OR later'*, or in the *'is it worth getting my help for my parents'*, you are essentially struggling with *'how important or unimportant is my (or my parent's) health?'*. Let us start by addressing the two major changes in hearing healthcare in the past decade.

#1. HEARING LOSS IS A PROGRESSIVE DEGENERATIVE DISORDER.

It wasn't long ago that most people in healthcare looked at hearing loss as a *nuisance* or something that was a *'normal part of aging'*. In fact, some people (thankfully not many!) still think of treating hearing loss as 'elective healthcare'—which implies that hearing is somehow a luxury that we can live without.

BUT THAT WAS THEN.

In the past decade, we have learned that hearing loss increases the risk of:

- dementia
- falls (#1 cause of injury-related death in adults)
- hospitalizations
- losing your home
- institutionalizations
- lost wages
- premature death!

I'm not trying to scare you, rather, I believe we are ethically bound to each patient to level with them and tell them what we know to be true and what research tells us every day.

SIGNS OF HEARING LOSS

- ringing in your ears
- blaming background noise for not being able to follow the conversation
- thinking *EVERYBODY* mumbles
- memory loss
- headaches
- loss of sleep
- desire to isolate (because being around others is not as enjoyable anymore!)
- feelings of embarrassment and guilt

Treating hearing loss and tinnitus is **not** elective healthcare. Hearing is medically necessary for healthy *social, emotional, physical,* and *cognitive* function. Allow me to briefly explain each one of these so that throughout the book you have a solid foundation of the medical benefits:

Social Health

Most often referred to as our ability to interact, form and maintain meaningful relationships. The majority of empirical research on hearing loss has a focus on the social impacts of this debilitating disorder.

Withdrawal from social situations is common in individuals with hearing loss, even in the earliest stage of the disorder. Most patients mention feelings of embarrassment, loneliness, inadequacy, fear of making mistakes in conversations, and feeling like they are not part of the conversation. Below is a quote from one of the most famous and brilliant composers that dates to the early 1800s. Unfortunately, I hear similar emotions from my patients in the 21st century.

> *"...my ears buzz and hum all the time, day and night. I may tell you that I lead a wretched life. Over the past two years I have avoided almost all social contact because I can hardly say to people 'I am deaf'."*
>
> —Ludwig van Beethoven

Fortunately, the data and real-life everyday experiences of my patients affirm that treating hearing loss and tinnitus improve quality of life and contribute enormously to their 'active aging'. We all share the same goal to maintain autonomy and independence as we age, and thus we must rely on preserving the tenets of interdependence (*socialization and reliance on family and loved ones*) and intergenerational solidarity (*maintaining companionship with age-matched peers*) to insure active aging.

Physical Health

It does not take an advanced degree to understand that physical activity is a requirement of maintaining proper health, especially as we age. But not everybody comprehends that untreated hearing loss results in people being less physically active.

Here is a fascinating statistic. Centenarians--people who live to be 100 years young or more--embody a fairly small percentage of the total U.S. population. In fact, only approximately 1 out of every 10,000 Americans are 100 years or older. This small slice of the population who are surviving to extreme old age lures the attention of not only researchers but also the public, as we attempt to recognize and learn from the experiences of those who beat the odds of environmental and biological hindrances to which most of us tend to fall prey.

Why do some people live such long, fulfilling lives, while others do not? Good question! Your first thought may be '*perhaps these individuals are genetically unique*'. The truth is genetics only play a 25% part in their endurance. Guess what the other 75% is? **Lifestyle & Activity!!** Ergo, we must remain active.

Emotional Health

Having positive emotional health is a fundamental aspect of healthy aging. In general, people who are emotionally healthy are in control of their thoughts, feelings, and behaviors. They are able to cope with life's challenges. They can keep problems in perspective and bounce back from setbacks. They feel good about themselves and have good relationships. That is not to say that people who are emotionally healthy are always happy and free from negative emotions, rather they have the skills to be able to manage the ups and downs of day-to-day life.

*But...*the amount of published research that details the negative impact of untreated hearing loss on emotional health, stress, anxiety, and depression is exhaustive. And the cost to manage these comorbidities (i.e., additional disorders that result from living with untreated hearing loss) is tremendous—both in terms of real dollars and in emotional bank. The medical treatment of hearing loss is one key ingredient to emotional health by strengthening social connections, helping increase quality of sleep, being mindful, and increasing self-esteem.

Cognitive Health

Perhaps the easier way to put this is: *living to a good age and having a good memory*. Like your brain, your ears never sleep. This means your brain is constantly stimulated by the vast neural network from your ears. ***Until it is not***. Then what happens?

Activities which stimulate the mind, *i.e., hearing*, can slow cognitive decline. What starts out as subtle cognitive changes that are seemingly associated with aging, go on to affect an older adult's day-to-day function. As we age, there are certain expected (albeit minor) cognitive changes that we will all experience. However, with increased risk of cognitive decline and dementia that may be the result of hearing loss, it is important to know the differences of 'normal aging', MCI (mild cognitive impairment) and dementia.

Early stages of significant cognitive decline (first seen in MCI) include problems with memory, language, thinking, judgement, and visual perception. Fortunately, most people are still 'with it' enough to notice these issues and can seek early intervention. Family and close friends may also notice a change. But these changes often are not severe enough to significantly interfere with daily life.

MCI along with hearing loss can increase your risk of later developing dementia caused by Alzheimer's or other neurological conditions. However, undeniable research is finding that early intervention of hearing loss improves cognitive function, including memory recall, processing speed and selective attention.

The medical treatment of hearing loss and tinnitus is the #1 modifiable factor for preventing dementia.

As we age, failure to spend even $5,000 on the medical treatment of hearing loss and tinnitus can easily create an $8,000 problem (the average cost to treat anxiety and stress), $30,000 (the average cost a family incurs when an older adult falls) or even a $57,000 per year problem (the average cost, *per year* to manage a loved one with dementia!).

You cannot stop your genetics from causing your hearing loss (and it is not worth getting mad and blaming your parents!). You also cannot go back in time and NOT attend that loud concert or perhaps take back all those years you spent working in a factory or restaurant, serving in the military, mowing the lawn, or playing in a band. THE DAMAGE IS DONE—and it will only get worse without treatment.

All it takes is finding the right hearing healthcare provider to truly "fix" your hearing loss and tinnitus and all the associated cognitive needs. Here is what I am told by so many patients and family members:

- *I am sorry I did not do this sooner.*
- *I had no idea how my hearing loss was impacting everybody around me.*
- *I wish I never let finances get in my way!*
- *This is SO EASY!*

#2. AGING ISN'T WHAT IS USED TO BE.

It wasn't too long ago that aging and retired adults spent most of their days in their homes and did not live an active lifestyle. I can vividly remember my grandmother in her house dress and my pop spending most of his days sitting in his chair. In less than a generation, there has been a dramatic change in how adults age. Older adults are working longer and *playing* longer! Heck... my 70-something year old mother wears jeans and Ugg boots; and she has a much fuller social calendar than I do!

Here are some **myths** about aging that we have all heard:

- People slow down with age.
- You can only learn new things when you are young.
- It is time to rest now.
- DECLINE IS INEVITABLE!

Here are some **truths** about aging (just to name a few!):

- Older adults who continue to challenge themselves with complex mental activities can delay or even reverse the normal decline in brain mass that is a part of primary aging.

- We are living longer (life expectancy has more than doubled in the past 120 years or so).

- In the U.S., the average 65-year-old male is expected to live to 80. If you reach 80, your life expectancy increases to age 90!

- The average 65-year-old woman in the U.S. is expected to live to age 85. Once she reaches 85, her life expectancy exceeds 90!

- Older adults who spend more time interacting with a wide range of people are more likely to be physically active and have greater emotional wellbeing.

- DECLINE IS OPTIONAL.

The fact is, your 50's, 60's, 70's, 80's and even 90's are your most formative years and set the course for how you want to be remembered and the legacy you leave. 'The back 9 of life', as my father referred to it, is your time to shine, your time to enjoy, your time to make the most of life.

THE TOP 5 REASONS PEOPLE AVOID SEEING THE HEARING CARE SPECIALIST

1. Patients are afraid/embarrassed/see it as a sign of aging.

Fear is the #1 reason most people avoid treating their hearing loss. Whether it be 'fear of the unknown', 'fear of costs' or 'fear of looking old', nearly 42 million people live with fear of accepting and treating their hearing loss and therefore do nothing about it.

Feelings of shame, inadequacy, being forgotten about, frustration, loneliness and insecurity are common in older adults with hearing loss. Often, people will deny themselves medical treatment for fear of being seen as 'old' by others. Trust me when I say this—not treating your hearing loss, not being part of the conversation, always saying '*what?*' and '*huh?*' when others speak—*that makes you look old!* (Sorry to be so blunt.)

2. Patients are afraid it is going to cost too much.

When it comes to treating hearing loss and tinnitus, much has changed in the past decade. Perhaps the biggest change is the *increase* in access and *decrease* in costs!! New treatment options for addressing hearing, tinnitus and associated cognitive decline are simple and affordable ***for all***. Our practices offer membership programs that make treatment affordable. Fortunately, gone are the days of having to pay large out-of-pocket costs. (If you are only given the option to pay for your treatment in full upfront—*run* the other way!).

3. Patients are afraid it is going to take too long/ miss too much work.

We understand that time is of the essence. Modern technology and ease of access allow us to work around your schedule AND be efficient with your time. We believe that time is of the essence, no matter your age. Modern technology used in most hearing healthcare offices allows for efficient diagnostic and treatment processes to make the most of your time in the office.

4.   Patients don't see the need to take action.

Untreated and *under*treated hearing loss (i.e., people who use traditional hearing aids or over-the-counter hearing aids) can significantly decrease their quality of life and increase their risk of dementia, falls, isolation, and premature death. In fact, not properly addressing your hearing loss and tinnitus can lead to a loss of independence. If you have early signs of hearing loss and tinnitus—you need to act, NOW!

5.   Patients have been treated in the past and it didn't work.

Let's face it, ***not all hearing healthcare specialists are created equal***. Every profession has its 'bad apples' and to say that audiology is an exception would be to write a tail of fiction. There is NO ROOM to be indifferent when it comes to choosing the right hearing healthcare provider. Finding the right practice means that they offer state of the art technology and state of the art service! The right provider offers every opportunity for patients to feel comfortable, safe, and having made the right decision (which is why our practice offers a *Lifetime Guarantee*—more about this in Chapter 9).

PREVENTING DECLINE

WE BROUGHT IN OUR 80-YEAR-OLD MOM, WHO STILL DENIED having hearing loss, for an evaluation. Our family was noticing changes and could tell that she wasn't going out as much and was isolating herself at home. We were beginning to be concerned with dementia setting in! Dr Darrow and his staff changed her life for the better!

We couldn't be happier after her treatment began. Within the first week she began going to dinner with friends again and playing cards with her social group every evening! You can't believe what a difference it made, it was honestly life changing! What a relief it was to know that being tested and treated for hearing loss wasn't our biggest fear of dementia, but simply hearing loss which is 100% treatable!

To Dr Keith and all the staff . . . THANK YOU for MAKING A DIFFERENCE and going above and beyond in treating our Mom with special care! We are forever grateful and a patient for life!

Donna O.
Patient at Hearing & Brain Center, Massachusetts
Excellence In Audiology Member

PREVENTING DECLINE

CHAPTER 2

WHY MUST WE TREAT HEARING LOSS & TINNITUS?

Is treating hearing loss nothing more than a great conspiracy (like Disney always trying to squeeze money out of patrons)?

Then, and now, there may be some overprescribing or even premature prescribing by some hearing healthcare providers (remember—there are bad apples in every orchard!)

But there is a very legitimate, clinically documented, medically approved, and 90+ percent of the time, clearly visible reason why some adults, sometimes as young as their 40s, *need* treatment and care: tinnitus.

Tinnitus (pronounced tin-ni-tus or tin-night-us; either is correct!), is most often, more than 90% of the time, attributed to the progressive and degenerative loss of nerves connecting the ear to the brain, (*aka HEARING LOSS*). Tinnitus is really just the fancy-pants word for 'ringing in your ears' or 'ringing in your head'. Ironically, people with hearing loss are often described as 'suffering in silence', when in fact, that is exactly the opposite of what most people with hearing loss deal with, as the tinnitus can severely impact living.

Simply put, as the nerves break down (from aging, genetics, noise exposure, medications, virus, etc.,) the brain will automatically make up for the missing signal and create the *false* perception of sound. This 'central gain' of neural activity can be altered with treatment (aka neuroplasticity), and therefore reduce the experience of tinnitus. The patients treated in our practice have tremendous success in reducing and/or eliminating their tinnitus. Chances are, when we begin your treatment, you have an 80+% chance of living with less (or no) tinnitus. While I am not much of a gambler... *I like those odds!*

If you or your loved one are suffering from any, several, or all of the following early indicators of hearing loss and tinnitus, consider having them addressed by a hearing healthcare specialist sooner rather than later:

1.   Noises in Your Ears or Head

Tinnitus is the internal alarm letting you know something is wrong. If left untreated, it **will** get worse. Tinnitus can interrupt your sleep, cause headaches and increase stress and frustration.

2.   Difficulty Hearing Others

Being left out of the conversation can be frustrating and embarrassing. Trust me, the more you 'smile and nod' your way through a conversation, the more people look at you and think 'wow, *she/he is getting old*'.

3.   Memory Issues

It is now considered medical truth that hearing loss can increase the risk of cognitive decline and dementia by as much as 200-500%, depending on degree of hearing loss. This means that even a "mild" hearing loss (which, I believe, is a really foolish term used to describe hearing loss—more on this in Chapter 7!) can increase the risk of dementia by 200%. Early signs that hearing loss and tinnitus may be impacting your memory include:

- memory loss that disrupts daily life (i.e. your spouse or children are getting mad at your for not remembering things)

- challenges in planning or problem solving (i.e. getting more confused that you normally do)

- difficulty completing familiar tasks (i.e. not completing your tasks and 'to-do' lists)

- confusion with time or place (i.e. losing track of time and location)

- problems identifying words and names (i.e. 'what was her name again?'

- misplacing things (i.e. losing your car keys way more than you should!)

- difficulty retracing steps (i.e. *wait a minute, how did I get here?!?!*')

- withdrawal from others (i.e. *'nah, I'd rather stay in than go out with friends'*")

- changes in mood and personality (i.e. becoming more frustrated and anxious than you ever used to be)

If you notice any of these signs in yourself or your loved one, **do something about it, *today*!** The right hearing healthcare provider understands the importance of early intervention, or as I most often say to patients, *'you have to catch it early and treat it early'*. The right hearing healthcare provider can help you understand the implication of cognitive decline, help you address how your hearing loss is playing a role in your decline, help you understand the other 11 risk factors of cognitive decline and dementia, and help you with additional resources.

The first question then is: *Do you have or show all the signs of early hearing loss, a progressive degenerative disorder?* Second, *if so, what should be done about it?* Third, *when?*

To answer all of these questions, the first comprehensive audiology exam should occur at 50 years of age. I passionately believe in the expression 'Ears and Rears'—the two things you must get checked when turning 50 years young. With early and periodic audiology exams, you may avoid the dire consequences of living with untreated hearing loss, the extra costs of living with untreated hearing loss, and living without the embarrassment and frustration related to untreated hearing loss. And don't forget, mid-life treatment of hearing loss is at the top of the list of ways which you can prevent dementia.

Waiting will have profoundly serious consequences, often requiring more treatment, higher costs, and ***poorer prognosis***! What too many patients fail to realize is that the signs of hearing loss are urgent and should be treated as such. I often say to patients 'the time for treatment is *yesterday!*' If you or your loved one need medical treatment of hearing loss—now or at some predictable future time—the outcome of the initial exam can help lead to more sensible decisions.

Let me be empathetically clear. I am **not** in the business of treating hearing loss for people who do not need it. My office is **not** a hearing aid store.

I *am* in the business of helping people and their families: obtain the right medical treatment of hearing loss and tinnitus if needed, access treatment, make treatment affordable, and hear and live their absolute best. *I believe the best patient is the educated patient.* In my offices, you are never told what to do. You are provided with real information, no medical jargon, plain English, the 'reasons why' you have hearing loss and tinnitus, and what your treatment options are.

Every adult with hearing loss and tinnitus needs treatment. But not all treatment is created equal. Together, we (you and I) will collaborate to figure out what is, or is not, needed, and what options are the best. And we will ***never compromise***.

PREVENTING DECLINE

HEARING LOSS HAS DEFINITELY TAKEN A TOLL ON MY DAILY life and I knew something needed to be done. I was fortunate to come to Dr. Darrow's practice where the staff provided me with knowledge, support, and treatment. Starting treatment has changed my life. The entire team did an amazing job highlighting the risk of dementia associated with hearing loss, knowing she had my best interest in mind. It was important for me to learn that treating hearing loss is not just for hearing health, but brain health. We evaluated my family history along with my loss and we began treatment immediately (and every question I had was answered). They were enthusiastic, passionate, and knowledgeable about treating hearing loss and was able to give me the individualized treatment that you can't find anywhere else!

Erin B.
Patient at Hearing & Brain Center, Massachusetts
Excellence In Audiology Member

CHAPTER 3

WHY NOT JUST ASK YOUR PRIMARY CARE? WHY A HEARING HEALTHCARE SPECIALIST?

You undoubtedly already have a primary care physician (even if you don't see her/him often enough!).

- *"But isn't seeing a hearing specialist going to cost me more?"*
- *"I'm busy."*
- *"More appointments?"*
- *"Do I really need to get regular audiology check-ups?"*

All reasonable questions.

It is true that, today, quite a few primary care doctors dance over into our territory (and even into other territories), and although the primary care doctor is a great centralized person to review *all* of your medical records, when you need specialty care, you need to seek a specialist. As an example, anybody reading this who has a heart condition or diabetes will absolutely have a cardiovascular and endocrinology specialist, respectively.

Specifically, those who specialize in hearing healthcare have additional training in the diagnosis and treatment of auditory conditions, including:

- presbycusis (age-related hearing loss)
- noise-induced hearing loss
- Meniere's disease
- tinnitus
- unilateral deafness
- sudden-onset hearing loss
- auditory neuropathy
- vestibular schwannoma

These are NOT primary care issues.
They are hearing healthcare issues.

There are some things for which a generalist or 'jack-of-all-trades' will do. For other things, you know it is smart to seek out the best specialist there is. Similar to the example provided above, when a patient is dealing with the dreaded cancer diagnosis, you do **not** want them to be under the care of a generalist. This is not to take anything away from all that a generalist has achieved and can do, rather it is to say that a generalist has no business treating cancer. Sorry, not sorry. I often think of the generalist in medicine as the 'general contractor' (G.C.) in construction. The best G.C. knows his/her limits and always hires the best electrician, the best carpenter, the best plumber, etc.

To elaborate—If all of your income is on a single W-2 from one employer and you have simple ordinary deductions, getting your taxes prepared for the cheapest fee at the seasonal tax office that opens in your neighborhood shopping center is probably fine (heck, maybe you can even do it yourself!). But, if you have W-2, 1099, investment income from real estate, depreciation on real estate in several states, own stocks and own a Christmas tree farm, you are going to need a *really* good accountant, i.e., a C.P.A.

Or let's say you need a simple will—leaving everything to your surviving spouse or only child is very straightforward. But, if you are of some means and have a few children, grandchildren, charities you support, investments, you are going to need to see a specialist: an estate planning attorney (not just *an* attorney).

Hearing healthcare is **no** different.

While these analogies have driven home my point, it is important to note that the same goes for your healthcare. When you suffer with the symptoms of hearing loss, including tinnitus, social isolation, memory loss, difficulty following a conversation, frustration, etc., you need a specialist. When you have hearing loss, a progressive degenerative disorder that impacts your social, emotional, physical, and cognitive health, you need a specialist.

Now that I have (hopefully) convinced you of the need to see a hearing healthcare specialist, now I have to help guide you on how to pick the **RIGHT** hearing healthcare specialist.

First, do they focus on the medical treatment of hearing loss, or do they just sell hearing aids? It does not take a special degree or a lot of money to open up a hearing aid shop. When you are searching for a hearing healthcare specialist, make sure you understand their credentials and medical affiliations. As a general rule of thumb, if the practice you are visiting is Excellence In Audiology™ approved, you are in the right place!

Second, is the medical treatment plan focused on treating your hearing loss and tinnitus, reducing your risk of dementia, maintaining your independence, decreasing your risk of falling, maximizing cognitive stimulation, and increasing your overall quality of life.... or do they just sell hearing aids? Unfortunately, the letters that come after somebody's name do not tell the full story. I've been in hearing healthcare for 20 years, and I have seen many 'bad apples' that are doctors of audiology, board certified hearing specialists and audioprosthologist. When a provider offers an inexpertly applied, standardized solution, they tend to be cheaper than the fees of a specialist that offers custom treatment plans. Cheaper, in hearing healthcare, implies there is an economic pressure on them to do treatment as quickly and as simply as possible, because they've 'cut it thin'. Cheaper, in hearing healthcare, also means that treatment outcomes may be compromised.

In this case, it is worth remembering that the medical treatment provided for hearing loss has permanent, lifelong, and life-impacting consequences. This concerns your health, including your risk of dementia, risk of falls, your ability to feel accepted and socialize with others, career longevity and your ability to be independent of others.

Healthcare Providers

- **Primary Care Doctor.** A healthcare professional that practices general medicine.

- **Ear, Nose and Throat Doctor (Otolaryngologist).** A person who has special training in diagnosing and treating diseases of the ear, nose, and throat.

- **Neurotologist.** A board-certified otolaryngologist who specializes in the surgical care of patients with diseases of the ear, temporal bone, skull base, head, and neck.

- **Audiologist.** A hearing healthcare professional who specializes in the diagnosis and treatment of hearing loss and balance disorders.

- **Hearing Instrument Specialist.** A person who is trained to diagnose, treat, and monitor disorders of the hearing and balance system.

When possible, you always want to choose a clinician who specializes in the treatment of your hearing loss and tinnitus.

You may ask, *'how do I know if my hearing healthcare provider is an audiologist or hearing specialist?'* It's a great question and a critical one to ask as you seek treatment for your hearing loss and tinnitus.

Only audiologists and hearing specialists that are qualified to be a member-clinic of the **Excellence In Audiology™** network can be found online at ***ExcellenceInAudiology.org***. You can find an approved specialist in your area that focuses on the medical treatment of hearing loss.

Alternatively, you can ask your hearing care provider if she or he has completed a fellowship in audiology or if they underwent the training to become a board-certified hearing specialist. You can also check with your state licensing board.

Do your homework; be a "hearing detective" while on the hunt for such vital information. Look for the words "medical treatment of hearing loss" or ask your generalist for a referral to a hearing healthcare specialist (not someone who just sells hearing aids!). In urban and suburban areas, it will take minimal effort to find a specialist. In more remote, rural locations, your search might take you to another city or town. Do not be afraid to travel for the best healthcare—**you are worth it**.

Side note: there is no disrespect between hearing healthcare providers and primary care/generalist providers. As a matter of fact, many audiology patients are referred by their PCP. These are great, capable, and caring professionals who know where their expertise begins and ends and do not let ego or income opportunity step in front of what they know is best for their patient.

Just as the generalist doctor must refer her/his patients with possible or significant heart disease to the cardiologist, and if need be, the cardiologist refers to the cardiovascular surgeon, the best generalists refer patients with audiology needs to the hearing healthcare specialist.

Hearing healthcare providers specialize.

THE QUALITY OF CARE PROVIDED BY THE ENTIRE STAFF IS SEC-
ond to none. Everyone in the office truly takes the time to listen to
the patient's needs and make sure s/he gets the best and most appropriate care available. Dr. Stirland, in particular, is one of the kindest,
most compassionate doctors I have seen for my hearing loss. I highly
recommend Intermountain Audiology.

Lisa H.

Patient at Intermountain Audiology, Utah (Cedar)
Excellence In Audiology Member

IT ALL STARTED WITH A WONDERFUL CONVERSATION WITH
Kathleen. She was extremely personable and patient with all my questions. We were greeted with aloha as soon as we stepped into office.
They were very hospitable and treated my mom well. Dr. Nakamura
catered to my mom's needs and was very thorough in explaining the
visit and the next steps.

James K.

Patient at Family Hearing Center, Hawaii
Excellence In Audiology Member

PREVENTING DECLINE

CHAPTER 4

CHOOSE A HIGHLY SUCCESSFUL HEARING HEALTHCARE PRACTITIONER

Why is that important? Wouldn't you get a "better deal" from one barely getting the light bill paid? Maybe. But an over eager hearing aid widget pusher might be seeing needs that are more urgent than they really are.

WHAT ARE SOME GOOD CLUES TO SELECT A GREAT HEARING HEALTHCARE PRACTITIONER?

I have got two: One, **she/he is busy**. Two, **her/his practice is busy**.

I assure you, the ability of advertising to attract patients is limited and it is expensive. When you see a really, really, busy practice there are probably a whole lot of patient referrals. Let's face it—nobody enthusiastically refers if they feel they were lied to or treated badly, sold something they did not need, and put their prescription technology in their underwear draw. And they probably wouldn't come to that practice if they had to keep coming back to 'fix a few things' or were overcharged. People only tell other people about their great experiences when they have their trust earned and when they have a truly unique experience.

I keep my offices very busy. Yes, we do some marketing. But mostly, our practices thrive by patient referrals. Not that I would anyway, but I do not need to wrangle you into more expensive care than you need to get the best outcome. I do not need to "sell" four more sets of hearing aid widgets this month to win a cruise from the manufacturer—and yes, that stuff goes on in some practices! There's an old cartoon from *The Wall Street Journal* with a bunch of executives in a boardroom at a conference table, one hollering, "Ethics? Ethics? We can't afford ethics!"

This is a business built on ethics and earned trust. And you do not just need a doctor to sell you some widget; you need an honest, trusted advisor.

The other clue: **a great hearing healthcare specialist is not cheap.**

Our fees are calculated to allow for "**Cadillac + Care**" in every respect, to put no downward financial pressure on how we care for patients, and to never compromise a patient's care. We never settle for "*this is probably good enough.*"

If I were you, I would worry if I could find a specialist that is a lot cheaper anywhere else. If you do find one, know this: behind closed doors they are probably asking, "can we do this cheaper?". Is that the question you want discussed by your care team at every step of your treatment process?

There is both a science and art to this. My specialists and staff are all highly trained to produce state-of-the-art outcomes, nothing less. The specialist truly makes a difference. That is why I tell everybody to get a highly successful hearing healthcare specialist.

THE TOP TEN THINGS YOU SHOULD KNOW BEFORE CHOOSING A HEARING HEALTHCARE SPECIALIST.

This is something you want to be sure about. I have just suggested one big consideration: a highly successful practice. Here are ten more:

1. Are they a specialist?

Tools have never created the skill. They're simply a conduit teaming with education, talent, experience, and knowledge. Audiology tools have never made the audiologist, but when the best tools are in the hands of the best specialists, magic happens.

All hearing specialists should be licensed by the state in which they practice, but not all hearing specialists have taken the next step to become members of the Excellence in Audiology™ network. This organization of hearing health care specialists have both the state-of-the-art tools and proven knowledge to do more than sell you a traditional hearing aid—their comprehensive hearing and cognitive treatment programs improve your hearing and cognitive function so you can maintain your independence longer—that independence is priceless!

In order to be a part of this network, a hearing health-care specialist must be thoroughly trained and tested to demonstrate their knowledge of the auditory system, clinical skills, and judgment. In addition to finding a local Excellence in Audiology™ specialist, you might consider a specialist who understands the hearing and brain connection as 'treating hearing loss' was recently named the single most modifiable risk factor for the prevention of the mind-robbing disease of dementia.

Signs of a specialist:

- Excellence in Audiology Member
- Certified Dementia Practitioner
- Incorporates Cognitive Screenings into testing protocols
- Offers Comprehensive Hearing and Cognitive Treatment Programs; not just traditional hearing aids
- Treatment Programs include ongoing brain training exercises
- Treatment technology is updated over time; without additional fees!

2. Do they have a Medical Office (or a sales office)

For years, the profession of audiology has received a bad reputation for its focus on the sale of traditional hearing aids by former used-car salesmen. In the audiology world it is not hard to open a shop on a shoe-string budget and call yourself a 'hearing aid specialist'.

When determining your family's next hearing health care specialist, I recommend you understand the treatment philosophy and purpose of the founder or specialist. Take the time to research his/her office, treatment team, website, location, and online testimonials and reviews. During your research, be on the lookout for stand-a-lone location or a medical setting that was founded many years ago and has helped thousands of individuals in your community.

Medical-based offices will focus on the signs and symptoms of hearing loss and tinnitus, the detrimental impact of un-treated and under-treated health conditions. You will notice that medical-based offices include many free reports, books, videos and educational opportunities to learn more about you or a loved ones' condition. Remember, *the educated patient is the best patient*.

Sales-based offices will focus on the makes, models, and prices of their traditional hearing aid technologies. I often refer to these providers and offices as 'widget salesmen'. Be on the lookout for words like 'FREE Test-Drive', 'FREE Demo', or 'Try Before You Buy' will be on their sales materials and advertising. Remember, free is just another word for 'has no value'.

3. Do They Think Brain Health First?

It might seem strange and go against everything you were taught in pre-school, but we don't actually 'hear' with our ears. The ears are just a receptor of sound, which is then transferred to our auditory nerve, and finally into our brain, where the speech understanding and cognitive process of deciphering sounds into words takes place. As a neuroscientist who has worked in the lab for over a decade and seen up close how the system works, this comes naturally to me, but to many hearing specialists without formal training or membership in a community like the Excellence in Audiology network it is often overlooked.

While words like dementia, cognitive decline, cognitive overload, progressive degenerative disorders and auditory system damage might seem scary, rest assured a hearing specialist and his/her team who thinks 'Brain Health First' will undoubtedly be using these words when discussing your hearing and tinnitus symptoms with you. If your specialist is not using these words, or is focused on things like lifestyle charts, bluetooth, rechargeable batteries and TV adapters you will know they are thinking 'hearing aids first' and not 'Brain Health First'.

Finding a local specialist who thinks 'Brain Health First' will make sure you and/or your loved one is not only improving your hearing, but also doing everything possible to reduce the increased risk of cognitive decline and dementia associated with hearing loss and auditory system damage. Treatment options from a 'Brain Health First' specialist will include the most modern hearing technology (sometimes called NeuroTechnology™) designed with the cognitive (brain) aspects of hearing loss in mind, including restoring the ability to hear in noise, filtering out background sounds, and boosting the soft-speech details needed to understand those around you.

Questions to ask:

1. What cognitive screening protocols do you use in your office?
Answers should include: "Cognivue," "Word Recognition Testing," and "Speech in Noise Testing"

2. Does your treatment plan include new treatment technology?
Answers should include: Our treatment plans only include new treatment technology (or NeuroTechnology™ . . . and never 'traditional hearing aids'

4.   Do They Provide Pre-Appointment Education?

Most traditional hearing aid sales offices will be in a hurry to get you right in for a "FREE Hearing Test". This is so they have the first chance to 'sell' you on their traditional hearing aid.

My recommendation is to find a medical-based office with a hearing health care specialist who goes out of their way to provide you pre-appointment education to help you and your family make the best decision on this major medical decision.

Some items I recommend requesting prior to your appointment:

- 7- to 14-day delay before your appointment to review all materials sent to you

- A book or publication by the practice owner or founder

- Any online presentations or educational materials available

- A detailed account of what is included in their comprehensive treatment program

- The cost of their all-inclusive monthly treatment plan

- What to expect during your first appointment

- It won't take you long to differentiate which office is focused on providing you education and conversation as opposed to looking to get you in as soon as possible.

5. Do They Offer Guarantees? If So, What Are They?

No matter which hearing specialist you choose, ultimately you are beginning a relationship with them. A relationship based upon a significant investment of both time and money to solve you or a loved ones' hearing loss or tinnitus problem. As with any relationship, it should be based upon trust and a guarantee that you will experience the expected outcome you are looking for.

The most common attempt at a guarantee in the field of hearing health care and audiology is a "traditional hearing aid return period." This is **NOT** a guarantee, this is a law required by every hearing healthcare specialist who is selling a traditional hearing aid widget.

When I speak of a 'guarantee' I am referring to the commitment of the founder, or owner, or hearing healthcare specialist you choose.

- *Do they guarantee your ability to hear will be restored to its full potential?*

- *Do they guarantee if you are unhappy at any point during the adaptation period you will part ways as friends and not spend a single penny for treatment received so far?*

- *Do they guarantee your hearing and tinnitus treatment is fully-covered with no additional fees during your treatment program?*

- *Do they guarantee that if at any time during your four-year treatment plan that if your hearing loss or tinnitus progressives severely enough that it requires a new prescription you will get that new prescription without increased monthly fees?*

- *Do they guarantee that your monthly cost of treatment will never increase due to rising costs or inflation?*

Now those are guarantees!

6. Are they Using the Latest Treatment Options Available?

Modern hearing loss diagnosis and treatment differs a great deal from years past. With the evolution of computer-designed technologies, hearing specialists with the proper equipment will be able to more accurately diagnose, treat, and improve your hearing and cognitive functions. Be on the lookout for a hearing specialist with modern technology and office vibe as opposed to someone who is stuck with antiquated technologies that will hold you back from living your best and healthiest life.

Modern technologies that should be used by a hearing specialist include:

- Speech in Noise Testing to determine your ability to hear in noise

- Cognitive Screening with Cognivue® Equipment

- New treatment technology that has artificial intelligence which focuses on restoring stimulation to the auditory system; improving hearing and reducing tinnitus

- Pre-and post-treatment testing to prove your results both in the testing booth and in background noise

- Audioscan Verfit2 Real-Ear Measurements to objectively measure the benefit of your new treatment

- Live-Speech Mapping to verify you are hearing all parts of the spoken language

- BrainHQ Brain Training Program for ongoing memory and processing speed improvements

7. Do They Offer a Comprehensive Treatment Membership?

Long gone are the days of spending thousands of dollars upfront on traditional hearing aids; *don't do it*!

Hearing loss is the third most common chronic condition affecting seniors in our communities. Like any major medical condition, the treatment of hearing loss, tinnitus and the associated cognitive impacts are not a one-and-done purchase of a hearing aid widget, but rather an ongoing monthly medical treatment. When you are searching for a hearing health care specialist, I recommend you find one who has a monthly treatment program or membership that allows you to begin treatment without investing thousands of dollars on day one.

An All-Inclusive Treatment Membership should include everything you need to properly treat your hearing and tinnitus, including:

1. Your prescribed hearing technology

2. Any supplies, accessories, or batteries you'll need

3. Coverage for loss or damage at a low deductible

4. All of your office visits and annual evaluations

5. Yearly cognitive/dementia risk screenings

6. And other various benefits:

    ▪ Early access to events

    ▪ Birthday gifts

    ▪ Special New Release education materials

    ▪ Supplements

    ▪ BrainHQ

7. A price lock guarantee so you don't have to worry about price increases in the future

## 8.	Do you get a direct phone number for 24/7 support or questions?

Hearing is 24/7, and so should your support line.

Each time a patient embarks on the journey of improved hearing or reduced tinnitus, there is an adaption period for the patient and their family. This period can take up to 60 days (perhaps longer for the most difficult cases of tinnitus) and is unique to each patient. Whether you or your loved one have a simple question, or need reassurance, your hearing health care specialist should give you a direct number to a patient experience coordinator just in case.

In addition to the complex hearing and cognitive changes that will happen as we begin restoring the stimulation to your auditory system, there can be moments of minor irritation or discomfort similar to wearing a new pair of shoes or prescription eyeglasses. Whatever question or concern you have, don't hesitate to ask!

A medical-based hearing health care specialist will provide you the means for direct support, as well as an established new treatment plan consisting of 3-4 appointments during the first 45-60 days of treatment. You should plan to visit your specialist 4 times per year for ongoing maintenance, re-evaluations, and prescription updates in addition to any fun or interactive patient events they may offer.

Remember, you should not have to pay additional fees or costs for this direct phone number, visits, patient events or ongoing hearing health care. It should be included in your comprehensive monthly treatment plan.

9. Do They Make You Feel Special and Comfortable?

Regardless if you are reading this report for your own hearing loss or tinnitus treatment, for a spouse, or another family member, you are the most important part of the health care practice.

The best hearing health care specialists, practices, and teams would be wise to remember that without the patient they would not have careers. As I've traveled the country speaking, educating, and working with private practices I continue to teach based upon the principles of Disney Magic, the Ritz Carlton Gold Standard, and the empathy found at the Cleveland Clinic.

When you walk into your new hearing healthcare specialist's office, you should be made to feel comfortable and welcomed. Empathy, compassion, and understanding are very important to the healing process.

Here are some things I recommend you should receive:

- Pre-Appointment Information
- Welcome Gift
- A Great look, feel, and smell to the office
- A Big Thank You
- Treat or Drink
- Walked to Your Treatment Room
- They should get to know you the person
- Understand your symptoms and desired outcome

- A Fond Farewell to Return

If you'd like the feedback of others prior to booking an appointment, try visiting their online views or video testimonials to learn more about what to expect at your appointment.

10. Do They Have a Great Reputation?

"Trust; but Verify!"

When it comes to choosing a hearing health care specialist, I prefer no other phrase.

With the internet today, it is extremely easy to pull up ratings, reviews, and testimonials from other patients. Simply go to Google, Facebook, HealthyHearing, or Yelp and search for audiology reviews in your town. I would recommend choosing the hearing health care specialist with the most reviews at the highest rating. This gives me comfort in knowing that they are busy enough to get the most reviews, and great enough to earn that high 5-star reputation.

At the time of writing this report, every Excellence in Audiology™ member-clinic has the most 5-Star reviews in their city. No other network of hearing health care specialists even comes close to this number of reviews.

In addition, with the growth of YouTube, many practices now have a YouTube channel full of real-life patients on video giving their own personal testimonial about the hearing health care specialist and office. So, remember, trust that your research has fulfilled the first nine questions of this report, but don't hesitate to verify with real patient review, testimonials and references.

And never be shy about asking for references- and go directly to the source! You have the right to call any hearing health care specialist and ask for a list of references who may be patients and/or local physicians who have volunteered to help advise other patients as they first enter the world of hearing loss and tinnitus treatment.

Okay, I know I said the list was only 10, but this last one is really important to consider!

11. Will They Make Treatment Affordable for Us?

I realize that I was only supposed to list the 'Top 10 Things You Must Know Before Choosing a Hearing Healthcare Specialist,' but I couldn't leave out some tips on making sure your choice of hearing health care specialist *never allows a treatment decision to become a financial decision.*

Once you are comfortable knowing the answers to the Top-10 questions and have chosen a hearing health care specialist to treat you, your spouse, or your loved one, the next questions is typically:

"Is this comprehensive treatment plan affordable?"

When it comes to affordability, there was no greater pain in my years as an audiologist than having to turn a patient away due to their financial situation. Thankfully our new treatment membership programs allow us to treat nearly every patient by reducing costs to a low, monthly, affordable payment. Your local Excellence In Audiology™ member-clinic will always offer an affordable membership plan to ensure that you don't have to make a treatment decision, or possibly compromise treatment, because of finances.

Benefits of Membership Based Hearing Healthcare:

- Avoid the Large Upfront Cost of Traditional Hearing Aids.

- Low Monthly Membership Plans for the Medical Treatment of Hearing Loss and Tinnitus

- All-Inclusive Coverage for your Hearing and Tinnitus Treatment Needs

- Price Lock Guarantee so Your Treatment Costs Won't Increase Over Time

- No Patient is Denied the Care they Need due to Bad Credit/No Credit

Remember to ask your local hearing health care specialist if they offer treatment membership programs to make your treatment more affordable.

How to Know What Questions to Ask

I have really thought through the questions most patients and family members ask — not just the ones they all ask, but also the ones they *do not* ask. This book attempts to cover them all, but overall, this is a *personal* matter. The best questions to ask are the ones that matter most to you and your loved ones.

I hope not—but you may be in a position absolutely requiring you to get the minimum essential treatment for the lowest cost. If so, your most important questions are going to be about those kinds of options and about price, and nothing else. However, I continue to recommend you find your local Excellence In Audiology™ member-clinic as they likely have a non-profit organization that may be able to help.

Below, I have included a *"What Is Most Important to You?"* quiz on the following pages. As you will see, there are fourteen different items to consider and rank in importance to you. Any of them can become the questions you ask me and my team or any other specialist.

Every practice that I work with takes a pledge of exceedingly high standards and we hold each other accountable. If you have a specific question not answered anywhere in this book, or have a personal and confidential question, you can—with complete assurance of privacy and courtesy—call your local member-clinic to discuss you or your loved one's needs.

There is also a FAQ section at the back of this book to help get you the answer you need.

Of course, a perfect opportunity to get questions answered—for you and your loved ones—is at your initial appointment.

Quiz: What is Most Important to You?

Directions: For each Key Item below, rank its importance to you from 1 to 5. Then check off whether each type of hearing healthcare specialist provides that item. When you're done with all 14 Key Items, add up your rankings and review what your final score means about choosing a hearing healthcare specialist.

Key Items to Consider in selecting your Hearing Specialist	Rank How Important Each Item Is To You in Selecting Your Hearing Specialist 1 - NOT Important, 5 - VERY Important	Check Off If Provided		
		Excellence In Audiology Members	Other Provider	Other Provider
1 Excellence In Audiology clinicians and staff are committed to expert, thorough diagnosis and prescription of the best treatment plan customized for myself or my family member	1 2 3 4 5	✓		
2 Avoiding Traditional Hearing Aids	1 2 3 4 5	✓		
3 Preventing loss of independence	1 2 3 4 5	✓		
4 Pain-free Treatment	1 2 3 4 5	✓		
5 Having healthy hearing that will cover all of my needs today and in the future	1 2 3 4 5	✓		
6 Hearing Specialist utilizes the most modern, advanced, and proven technology, including computer-aided prescriptions and stimulation	1 2 3 4 5	✓		
7 Hearing Specialist and team actively involved in continuing clinical education	1 2 3 4 5	✓		
8 Reducing treatment time to a minimum without compromising results (including number of office visits)	1 2 3 4 5	✓		

Key Items to Consider in selecting your Hearing Specialist	Rank How Important Each Item Is To You in Selecting Your Hearing Specialist 1 - NOT Important, 5 - VERY Important	Check Off If Provided		
		Excellence In Audiology Members	Other Provider	Other Provider
9 Availability of after-work appointment options	1 2 3 4 5	✓		
10 Treatment Coordinator is knowledgeable about insurance coverage and is able to offer simple and affordable treatment plans	1 2 3 4 5	✓		
11 Lifetime guarantee	1 2 3 4 5	✓		
12 Hearing Specialist and team committed to excellence in audiology and customer service for both patients and family members	1 2 3 4 5	✓		
13 No down-payment required	1 2 3 4 5	✓		
14 Avoiding cognitive decline, falling and disconnecting with others	1 2 3 4 5	✓		

Total of Your Rankings

What Your Score Means

50 to 70   There is no doubt. Your local Excellence In Audiology member-clinic is the right choice for you and your family! It is clear you place high value on a comprehensive "best" approach to the medical treatment of hearing loss and tinnitus

43 to 49   You are probably also going to be the happiest with your local Excellence In Audiology member-clinic, rather than any other alternative. But this score suggest you aren't completely sure and have some unanswered questions or concerns. Your Hearing Specialist and Treatment Coordinator want no lingering uncertainties on your part, and want to address any and every question. Don't keep anything to yourself. Please ask!

42 or less   Frankly, you may not value the advanced, sophisticated level of clinical care and service provided at Excellence In Audiology member-clinics. Cost may be much more important to you than other factors, or very basic service may be all you feel you need. As you shop around, I recommend you continue to use this checklist to evaluate all of your options and see what is best for you or your loved one.

PREVENTING DECLINE

HEARING? WE NEVER APPRECIATE THE VALUE OF GOOD HEAR- ing, until we lose that which we have always taken for granted. Similarly, we never appreciate a specially caring and talented clinician like Dr. Larry Cardano, without having experienced others.

Two things I have learned these thirty years:

Firstly; There is a huge difference between basic units (sold online and on TV), which are just amplifiers, and the state of the art units— powerful computers which are able to analyze, process and clarify sounds that you actually need to hear.

Secondly—and as important: I learned that an investment in quality hearing healthcare is worthless without the right clinician. Most quality hearing aids today don't receive the fine tuning that they need to work most effectively in the user's ears. You need a caring and concerned provider who will take the time over multiple visits—to micro tweak the numerous software controlled parameters that can make the difference between your hearing aids being a pleasure and them being a pain.

These complex units today also need firmware updates, spare parts and an understanding of how their automatic modes can be expected to work in various conditions so as to know how to anticipate their function and vary curves and sliders in the software to get them to do what both your ears and mind will need to make sense of the sounds you want to hear.

One's natural hearing will continue to decline as one ages. If you are an active person—or for anyone to whom hearing is important— you have to go to Dr. Cardano and his caring associates help you hear better.

Gary R.
Patient at Hearing Centers of Long Island, New York
Excellence In Audiology Member

PREVENTING DECLINE

CHAPTER 5

What Can I Expect at the Initial Consultation and Exam?

Many questions surround your first visit to a new hearing healthcare specialist, not the least of which is the subject of this particular chapter: *what will happen at the initial consultation?*

To answer this quite common question, and perhaps several others you might not even realize you need answering yet, let me walk you through the typical first office visit, from the initial appointment forward. Your first appointment is scheduled following your initial phone call to your hearing healthcare providers office.

1. **On arrival at the office, you will be greeted by one of our certified treatment coordinators.**

   She or he is fully prepared to make everything from the first appointment to the entire treatment program go smoothly for you and your loved one. Your treatment coordinator will be yours to manage your relationship with us, from appointment scheduling to answering questions.

At the initial visit, your treatment coordinator or provider will review your patient information and health history and address any concerns that you may have. For example, you will be asked questions like "why did you decide that today was the right day to start the treatment process?", "what do you know about the medical treatment of hearing loss and tinnitus?", "do you have concerns of dementia (and is there a family history of cognitive issues)?", "are you living with diabetes (or pre-diabetes)?", "have you fallen and/or are you concerned about falling?", etc. Each of these are critical to designing the right treatment plan.

2. Next, your hearing specialist will conduct a thorough evaluation.

The most complete and thorough audiology exam has three steps:

- **Step 1.** Assess your risk of cognitive decline.
- **Step 2.** Establish your degree of hearing loss.
- **Step 3.** Determine the impact your hearing loss is having on your cognitive function.

Given what we know about the strong links of hearing loss and dementia, performing Step 2 without Step 1 and 3 are essentially a waste of time. Unfortunately, many hearing offices still only perform step 2.

The same day, your hearing healthcare specialist will present their "findings and diagnosis". This will walk you and your family members through the stages of hearing loss (more to come on this in Chapter 7) and lay out the entire treatment plan. *Given how important this information is, we ask every patient to bring at least 1 family member with them to review the diagnosis and treatment plan.*

If treatment should occur, your hearing healthcare specialist will present recommendations and options. This will be an individualized, personalized plan of treatment. It will **not** be traditional hearing aids and it will not be 'one size fits all'.

Your audiology report must include the following:

- Current Stage of Hearing Loss (Stage 1 to 4)
- Dementia Risk Assessment
- Falls Risk Assessment
- Treatment Recommendation
- Treatment Prognosis (quantifiable and measurable)
- Recommendation for Follow-Up Testing

If you are handed a piece of paper that only has a graph on it (often called the 'audiogram') and are simply told 'you have a mild hearing loss and need a hearing aid', you are **not** getting all the information you deserve!

3.   All your questions will be answered.

There are no dumb or embarrassing questions—I believe in the old adage 'the only dumb question is the one not asked!'. Of the countless patients who have visited my office, every one of them had questions! We do not want you or your son or daughter just nodding, then later wondering, "what did he mean by that?" or saying "I wish I'd asked about ..." This is not one of those "I'm the doctor—trust me—just do what I say because I said so" offices. We hope that most questions are answered on the phone, by this book and by the materials we send to each patient who books an appointment. *BUT* we understand this can be a lot to take in and you may still have burning questions. Any and all questions you have should be asked and answered. As I've stated already in this book, I believe *'the best patient is the educated patient'*.

4. Your treatment coordinator or provider will explain the costs of the prescribed treatment program.

The medical treatment of hearing loss and tinnitus must be affordable *without* compromising treatment outcomes. Our practices have figured this out and our treatment membership plans help more patients afford treatment with a low monthly cost plan. (More on *How to Pay for the Medical Treatment of Hearing Loss and Tinnitus* in Chapter 11). As the saying goes, a journey of a thousand steps begins with the first one.

5. Finally—the reason you came in—we recommend starting treatment on Day 1.

The average patient waits 7-10 years before admitting they have a hearing loss and is willing to start treatment. The last thing we would make a patient do is wait any longer. Hearing loss is a major medical condition that impacts every aspect of a patient's life, including physical, social, emotional, and cognitive health. Ask any of the hundreds of students I have trained over the years and they will tell you—my favorite saying to my patients' is '*we need to begin treatment* **yesterday**'.

In total, you should allow about 1.5 hours for this entire initial consultation, exam, and to begin treatment.

If that seems like a lot of time, keep in mind there are a life-time of health benefits to proper hearing healthcare. This is not like "installing tires"— at least not when it is done properly and expertly. You and your loved one deserve a careful, thorough, and *anxiety-eliminated* experience.

Frankly, our practice and our process are not for everybody. We attract and "resonate with" patients and families who are quite serious about their commitment to health and self, and to their family. Our treatment plans are intended to keep social, physical and cognitive decline at bay, and keep patients confident and fiercely independent. If you are that patient, and the fact that you took the time to read this book suggests it, then you are going to recognize that this is time well invested in the best possible results.

PREVENTING DECLINE

I STOPPED INTO AUDIOLOGY ASSOCIATES LAST FRIDAY AT noon. They were prompt from the get-go. Both the assistant and the clinician were exceptional. They took whatever time I needed to explain to me the process and were very thorough in their evaluation. I have had pretty severe tinnitus for 15 years. Treatment has dramatically changed my life. Yes, it has a cost associated and yes, it is absolutely worth it! For the first time in many years I could actually clearly understand what people were saying to me, even in public areas with background noise. The cost is for a four year plan. Well worth it in my book.

Update: Here I am about six months from my initial fitting. I have been into the office several times to have adjustments made and make sure everything is working right. It always amazes me at how quickly my concerns are addressed and how immediately I am attended to. They are fantastic and it is obvious they get great pleasure with making sure that my life is better. Worth every penny!

James V.
Patient at Audiology Associates, Alaska
Excellence In Audiology Member

CHAPTER 6

Why You Must be Offered a Cognitive Screening for Dementia

Dementia is the single largest unaddressed public health threat in the 21st century and we must remain on the front lines of this crisis every day.

We all know a friend, neighbor or loved one who has been touched by Alzheimer's or dementia and understand the devastating toll this disease takes on families. I lost my grandmother, Mary Agnus Darrow, to dementia.

It has been nearly a decade since the first reports indicated a strong correlation of hearing loss and dementia. I have been an audiologist every day since this report first came out of Johns Hopkins in February 2011. I live, eat, sleep, and breath this knowledge every day. Since then, I have become the only National Certified Alzheimer's Disease and Dementia Care Trainer in the field of hearing healthcare. My practices started doing qualitative dementia screenings in our offices over 6 years ago. It was about 5 years ago we started offering patients the opportunity for genetic testing of known dementia-related genes.

And for the last three years we have been offering patients the opportunity to have an F.D.A-cleared (Food and Drug Administration) computerized test of cognitive function.

To put it lightly... I am obsessed with finding ways to help patients understand their dementia risk, improve their cognitive function, and take steps to prevent the disorders of dementia.

Every 3 seconds another person is diagnosed with dementia. That means, *in the time it takes you to read this sentence, another person has been diagnosed with dementia*. That is another person who has been handed down the diagnosis of *fatal brain failure*, another family that will have to pay the emotional toll of caring for a loved one at least 10 years beyond that person's mental capabilities. At an average cost of $57,000 per year to care for a loved one with dementia—it is also one of the costliest diseases on the planet.

Nearly 9 out of 10 older adults get their blood pressure checked when they visit their primary care doctors. Only 16% are even asked about problems with memory or thinking.

Our assessment tool, Cognivue™, is an important and innovative psychometric tool for cognitive evaluation. This test evaluates 6 cognitive domains: visuospatial, executive function/attention, naming/language, memory, delayed recall, and abstraction. With this tool, we also measure two speed performance parameters: reaction time and speed processing.

Every hearing healthcare practice in America *should* have a quantifiable means of assessing cognitive function and evaluating dementia risk. Here are two things we know, unequivocally:

1. Hearing loss is correlated with an increased risk of dementia by as much as 200-500% (depending on degree of hearing loss).

2. Four out of every 10 (or 40%) of people diagnosed with dementia are considered **PREVENTABLE**.

Perhaps the scariest medical statistic I have ever come across was from a survey of Medicare beneficiaries: *Half of Americans with Alzheimer's disease have not been diagnosed, and half of those with a diagnosis have not been told about it*. If you need to, please re-read that last sentence. Thankfully, new state laws are popping up all over our country that address this issue and require proper dementia training of most healthcare clinicians.

In 2017, the European Dementia Commission put forth the 'holy grail' on the state of dementia in our world. I will not bore you, or perhaps scare you, with the details, i.e., the overwhelming numbers of people who have dementia, the exponential increase in expected dementia diagnoses in the next 10-20 years, or all the things we do on a daily basis to increase our risk of dementia, but I will summarize how you can err on the side of caution and increase your chances of living a dementia-free life!

This report, published in the Lancet (FYI—the **Lancet** is among the oldest, most respected, and most widely read medical journals in the world) and recently updated in 2020 lays out the '*How To*' of preventing dementia.

NOTE: These 12 items are listed IN ORDER of percentage chance of avoiding dementia if this risk is eliminated:

1. **Hearing Loss**—The early medical treatment of hearing loss is *the* most modifiable lifestyle factor for reducing the risk of dementia.

2. **Increased Education**: Your mother was right—stay in school and never stop learning.

3. **Stop Smoking**: If the threats of lung cancer and emphysema are not enough to get you to stop smoking, perhaps ending up without dementia will.

4. **Depression**: Addressing depression in older age is critically important for cognitive health, and healthy hearing goes a long way to reducing depression.

5. **Social Isolation**: There is a reason that my first book title has the word 'isolation' in it—hearing loss is a major contributor to social isolation and withdrawal from friends and family. Treat your hearing loss and stop living in isolation.

6. **Traumatic Brain Injury (TBI)**: While most TBIs are the result of an accident, preventative measures should always be taken to reduce the incidence of TBI, therefore reducing the risk of dementia.

7. **Physical _Inactivity_**: People with hearing loss are less physically active. This has been shown time and time again in research and likely is the result of increased social isolation in older adults with hearing loss.

8. **Hypertension:** What is good for the heart is good for the mind! Cardiac conditions compromise blood flow to nearly all major organs, including the brain and the ear. Love yourself and take care of your heart.

9. **Air Pollution:** This was recently added to the list as air pollution might act via vascular and/or respiratory mechanisms and reduce proper blood and oxygen flow to the brain.

10. **Diabetes:** Several studies suggest that the brains of people with Alzheimer's disease are in a 'diabetic state', partly due to the decrease and insensitivity to insulin. Diabetics are at least twice as likely to experience dementia.

11. **Obesity:** Being overweight is an emerging concern when it comes to dementia. The rates of increased BMI in older adults are growing and may be contributing to cognitive decline.

12. **Alcohol Intake:** Like most things we enjoy in life, moderation is key. Consuming less than 21 units of alcohol per week (the equivalent of 2 bottles of wine per week) can help to reduce the risk of cognitive decline and dementia as we age.

Because I am obsessed with helping people prevent dementia, allow me to summarize the above findings of the Dementia Prevention, Intervention and Care Report (2020) two more ways:

1. Treating hearing loss is:
- *8 times* more effective at reducing your risk of dementia than reducing obesity
- *8 times* more effective at reducing your risk of dementia than reducing diabetes
- *4 times* more effective at reducing your risk of dementia than reducing hypertension
- *4 times* more effective at reducing your risk of dementia than increasing physical activity, and
- *2 times* more effective at reducing your risk of dementia than increasing social engagement with others.

2. Treating hearing loss is more effective at reducing your risk of dementia than if you reduce obesity, diabetes, alcohol consumption, and heart disease and increase physical activity, *combined!*

I hope this gets my point across. While I certainly cannot guarantee that if you do everything on this list that you will *not* get dementia, I do guarantee that you are doing everything you possibly can to reduce your risk of getting dementia.

Risk Factors For Dementia

The Lancet Commission on Dementia prevention, intervention and care has put forth a list of 12 modifiable risk factors to reduce the risk of Dementia.

Note that addressing hearing loss is the #1 most modifiable factor.

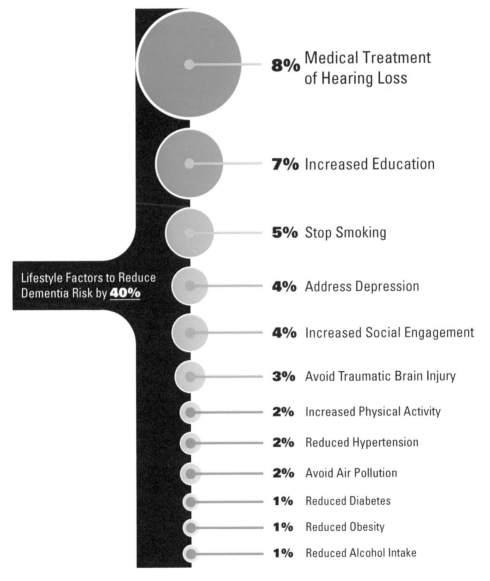

8% Medical Treatment of Hearing Loss

7% Increased Education

5% Stop Smoking

Lifestyle Factors to Reduce Dementia Risk by **40%**

4% Address Depression

4% Increased Social Engagement

3% Avoid Traumatic Brain Injury

2% Increased Physical Activity

2% Reduced Hypertension

2% Avoid Air Pollution

1% Reduced Diabetes

1% Reduced Obesity

1% Reduced Alcohol Intake

PREVENTING DECLINE

MY FIRST VISIT EVER TO AN AUDIOLOGIST AND THIS PLACE was fantastic, I was told on each test what to expect and when it came down to getting my hearing devices, Dr. Mistic made everything look so easy and when it was my turn to put my ear devices in, it was so easy. The people working in NewSound Solutions made you feel like they knew you forever, such a pleasant environment. I highly recommend if you are having hearing issues make an appointment and go you won't be disappointed.

Vicki G.
Patient at NewSound Solutions, Texas
Excellence In Audiology Member

I HAVE BEEN RELYING ON TIMPANOGOS HEARING FOR MY hearing needs for well over ten years and have experienced complete satisfaction with the care and concern they have shown me. Dr.Garrett is very knowledgeable and up-to-date on the technology and shares it freely. The support given me with my hearing needs over the years has been, and continues to be, unparalleled.

Ronald B.
Patient at Timpanogos Hearing & Balance, Utah (Salt Lake City)
Excellence In Audiology Member

CHAPTER 7

WHAT ARE THE STAGES OF HEARING LOSS?

If you or a loved one have hearing loss, you are probably used to hearing words like '*I lost 40% hearing in my right ear*' or '*my doctor told me I have a mild hearing loss*' or (my personal pet peeve) '*they said my hearing is normal for my age*'. Frankly—each of these is wrong. No member of the Excellence In Audiology™ hearing healthcare network should use any of these terms when describing hearing loss to a patient. And just to clarify—there is *no such thing as 'age-adjusted hearing loss'*— you either have hearing loss or you don't. There is no 'sliding scale' because of your age *and* there is no such thing as 'normal hearing loss'—that is an oxymoron.

Understanding your diagnosis is the first step in any successful treatment plan. Using terms like 'mild' or 'moderate' do not have much meaning. Additionally, making incorrect statements like '40% loss' does not help anybody and are inaccurate—until you are dead, and somebody goes poking around your ears and brain, a percentage should not be assigned to a hearing loss.

Like nearly all major medical conditions, a hearing loss diagnosis must be 'staged' to be best understood and to lay out realistic expectations and prognosis for treatment.

STAGE 1
Early stage hearing loss (15-40 decibels of loss) with some impact on cognitive function.

Patients with Stage 1 hearing loss are caught at the earliest phase of the disorder: thus, having the greatest prognosis for treatment. At this early stage, the hearing loss may be beginning to show early signs of impacting cognitive function with some impacts on memory recall and name finding.

Although many people living with this hearing loss may consider it *'just a nuisance'*, it is important to understand that hearing loss is a progressive degenerative disorder that can significantly increase your risk of dementia, falling, and a host of other co-morbid disorders.

Even at this earliest stage, these test results indicate marked damage to the nerves that connect the ear to the brain—which can have a host of downstream impacts, including tinnitus, difficulty following a conversation, and implication for memory loss and forgetfulness. Patient symptoms often include noticeable tinnitus (heard in the ears and/or head), subtle difficulty with details of speech (missing the beginning or end of what others are saying), some loss of environmental auditory awareness (i.e., difficulty hearing knocking at the door, the refrigerator, alarm, etc.). In addition, the person will notice conversation is becoming more difficult to follow in background noise (and when watching TV). Patients with Stage 1 hearing loss must be

applauded for not waiting and catching this destructive disorder early—before it can fully infiltrate and wreak havoc on the
brain.

Stage 1 hearing loss is correlated with a near 200% increased
risk of developing cognitive decline and dementia. While that
may be a shock to you, what is most important is to understand
that research indicates that the early treatment of hearing loss
can dramatically reduce that increased risk of dementia (and
slow the progression of the disorder). Also, Stage 1 hearing loss
significantly increases the risk of falling by 140% (the #1 cause
of hospitalizations in older adults). However, with treatment and
access to the entire auditory environment, this risk of falling de-
creases significantly.

Stage 2
Mid stage / significant hearing loss (40-70 decibel of loss) with noted impact on cognitive function.

Patients with Stage 2 hearing loss have most likely waited anywhere from 3-6 years before reporting their symptoms and deciding to act. Fortunately, for most patients with Stage 2, the
prognosis for treatment remains high. Although there is nota-
ble damage to the neural connections from the ear to the brain,
there remains enough treatable hearing to provide proper cognitive stimulation and overcome deficits in clarity, tinnitus, and
auditory deprivation.

Patients with Stage 2 hearing loss often report the following
host of symptoms: annoying tinnitus (sound heard in the ears
and/or head), difficulty hearing others (i.e., missing when somebody is speaking to you), lack of ability to hear environmental

auditory cues (i.e., difficulty hearing when people are walking towards you, safety alarms in the home, a grandchild crying from the other room). With this stage of hearing loss, it is a significant struggle to follow a conversation when with a group of more than 2 and in restaurants.

With Stage 2 hearing loss, the goal is to provide maximum neurocognitive stimulation, which the brain needs to run on all cylinders. In fact, if you do not mind sticking with the 'engine' reference, living with untreated hearing loss is like driving 60mph in second gear—which, over time will wear down the system and cause significant damage. The treatment of hearing loss can dramatically improve cognitive function—this has been shown in numerous studies and it is certainly something our patients have to look forward to!

Stage 2 hearing loss is correlated with a near 300% increased risk of developing cognitive decline and dementia. Again, what is most important is to focus on the positive—which is that research indicates that the early treatment of hearing loss can reduce that increased risk of dementia (and slow the progression of the disorder). Also, Stage 2 hearing loss significantly increases the risk of falling (the #1 cause of injury-related death in older adults). However, with treatment and access to the entire auditory environment, the risk of falling can decrease dramatically.

STAGE 3
Mid-late stage / severe hearing loss (70-90 decibels of loss) with significant impact on cognitive function.

Patients with Stage 3 hearing loss often wait the average 7-10 years before reporting their symptoms and seeking treatment.

While prognosis is still positive and a successful treatment plan is anticipated, hearing loss at this stage can begin to show a significant impact on cognitive function. At this stage, there is marked damage to the neural connections from ear to brain—which expand beyond the auditory centers and reach deep into the memory, sensory and emotional portions of the brain.

As a result of the neural damage, the patient will experience a myriad of symptoms, including bothersome tinnitus (sounds in the ears and/or head that interfere with hearing, sleep, etc.,), inability to hear what others are saying (even in a quiet environment), lack of ability to hear important environmental auditory sounds (i.e., difficulty hearing the phone, smoke / CO_2 alarms). At Stage 3 hearing loss, most patients will begin to avoid social gatherings and isolate themselves as they will not be able to converse and interact in a restaurant or any social setting with 2 or more people.

The auditory stimulation provided at this stage will focus on the areas with the most damage, as well as the portions of the brain that remain most active for hearing. Although individual prognoses may vary, outcomes will be positive and provide access to conversation, even in noisy situations.

Stage 3 hearing loss is correlated with an approximate 400% increased risk of developing cognitive decline and dementia. Although this may seem like a 'late stage', all research indicates positive outcomes that can work to reduce the risk of cognitive decline and dementia (and potentially slow the progression of the disorder). Also, Stage 3 hearing loss dramatically increases the risk of falling. However, even at this stage, with treatment and access to the entire auditory environment, the risk of falling can decrease.

STAGE 4
Late stage / profound hearing loss (90+decibels of loss) with substantial impact on cognitive function.

Patients with the most advanced stage of hearing loss will benefit from treatment. Period. Despite the significant neural and cognitive damage.

With many medical conditions, 'Stage 4' is often thought of as the 'untreatable' stage; *this does not apply to hearing loss*. At Stage 4, there is significant damage to nearly the entire hearing structure and the nerves that connect the ear to the brain. Fortunately, it is less often that we see a 'first-timer' patient who presents with Stage 4 on day one.

When left untreated this hearing loss is truly disabling to the person and family. At this point in the disorder, patients will experience symptoms that alter everyday life, including constant interfering tinnitus (sounds in the ears and/or head that make hearing, sleeping, etc. difficult) inability to hold a conversation with loved ones, lack of ability to hear life-threatening environmental sounds (i.e., inability to hear smoke / CO_2 alarms, emergency vehicles). Left untreated, patients with Stage 4 hearing loss will avoid social gatherings and isolate themselves as they are unable to interact with others.

Stage 4 hearing loss is correlated with a near 500% increased risk of developing cognitive decline and dementia. Although it may seem that all hope is lost at this stage, there are tremendous advances in recent technology that can help the person with the most profound degree of hearing loss to hear well again. All research indicates positive benefits of treatment that may reduce the risk of cognitive decline and dementia (and potentially slow the progression of the disorder). Also, Stage 4 hearing loss severely increases the risk of falling. However, even at this stage, with treatment and access to the auditory environment, the risk of falling can be decreased.

Always be sure that you understand your diagnosis and prognosis before moving forward with your recommended treatment plan.

I HAVE BEEN A PATIENT FOR MANY, MANY YEARS AND through major events in my life such as college, pregnancy, new baby, 9/11, hurricanes and now COVID-19. At this point, an appointment or phone call feels like talking to a beloved family member. Brooklyn Audiologist provides services with a person- centered approach. I feel valued, respected and my concerns are taken seriously. I don't have to wait long to schedule appointments or be seen when I am in the office. If my device needs to be repaired, I am given a loaner device in the interim to ensure that my everyday life will not be interrupted. As a mother and working professional with a demanding job, it was extremely important that my hearing and my devices are up to standard. I can rely on Brooklyn Audiologist and so can you.

Rosell B.
Patient at Brooklyn Audiology Associates, New York
Excellence In Audiology Member

PREVENTING DECLINE

CHAPTER 8

Understanding Your Hearing Disorder

Diseases and disorders of the ear come in all shapes and sizes, degrees, and stages. While the most common cause of hearing loss and tinnitus is aging, the truth is, it is not your age, rather it is your genes. Most of us will inevitably suffer with hearing loss as we get older, *not* because of working in noise or going to too many rock concerts (not that they make matters any better!), rather most species of mammals (including us) carry genes coded for age-related hearing loss. Presbycusis is the official medical jargon used by specialists when diagnosing this type of hearing loss.

The next most common cause of hearing loss is exposure to loud noises. Unfortunately, proper hearing health is not a common topic in most 'health classes', therefore the general public has no idea how noisy and how harmful most of our surroundings are. Another misnomer of hearing loss is that a 'hearing hangover' (i.e. when you go to a loud concert and your ears ring!) is something we can rebound from. Most scientists and clinicians once believed that this temporary ringing in the ears was something you could recover from and go right back to hearing normally. *This is not true.*

In the past 10-15 years, study after study has proven, over and over again, that these 'hearing hangovers' have a **permanent** effect on the auditory system and cause massive damage that cannot be recovered or healed. You might be saying to yourself *'is this for real.... my hearing was back to normal 2 days after that last wedding I went to.'* The facts are that the damage was real, but that the damage will not manifest itself in the form of de-tectable hearing loss for up to 2-3 decades (e.g. 20-30 years!). Hopefully, this has your attention now as you think back to all those loud restaurants you went to, the factory you worked in for 6 months, all the times you weed-wacked the lawn, and that rock band you were in when you were a teenager. When you combine your history of noise exposure (both big and small) plus your genetic predisposition to hearing loss as you age... you may have a perfect storm brewing that creates disabling hearing loss and tinnitus.

Rounding out the next most common forms of hearing loss and tinnitus are medication-induced, Meniere's Disease and sudden-onset. While most prescription drugs that impact the ears are necessary and life-saving/prolonging, many prescrip-tions have a side-effect of damaging cells in the ear (technical-ly it is called ototoxicity—meaning it is toxic to the ear). Strong antibiotics such as Ciprofloxacin can be damaging to the ear. Many chemotherapies used for the treatment of cancers have a component that is deadly to the cells in the ear. Even commonly available OTC drugs such as Aspirin and NSAIDS can increase the likelihood of developing hearing loss and tinnitus. And too much quinine (found in tonic water) can damage the ears too!

One of the most disabling causes of hearing loss, which presents with the triad of symptoms, i.e., hearing loss, tinnitus, *and* dizziness, is Meniere's Disease. The cause (or pathophysiology) of this disorder is the result of excess fluid trapped inside the inner ear. The overload of fluid will impact both the auditory and balance centers and send misguided information to the brain, rendering the patient deprived of sound input and the feeling of dizziness.

Currently there is no cure for Meniere's, but there are effective treatments available to alleviate the hearing loss and balance issues. Treatments include the following:

- **Medical Treatment of Hearing Loss and Tinnitus.** With advanced treatment technology, cognitive stimulation can restore sound, reduce the ringing, and provide auditory awareness to reduce the risk of falling.

- **Medications.** The most disabling symptom of a Meniere's Disease 'attack' is dizziness. Prescription drugs are available to relieve dizziness and shorten the attack.

- **Salt Restriction and Diuretics.** Limiting salt intake and use of diuretics (water pills) help some people control dizziness by reducing the amount of fluid the body retains, which may help lower fluid volume and pressure in the inner ear.

- **Nutritional & Dietary Changes.** Some people report that caffeine, chocolate, and alcohol make their symptoms worse and either avoid or limit them in their diet. Not smoking may also help reduce the symptoms.

"You know at first it was—suicical, tormenting . . . I have loud tinnitus, I lose my hearing, I realize I can't sing, I'm miserable, I'm lying in bed all day, I'm contemplating my demise. Horrible stuff, just awful."

—HUEY LEWIS DISCUSSING HIS
EXPERIENCE WITH MENIERE'S DISEASE

For most people who suffer with the instantaneous, life-altering, experience of **sudden-onset hearing loss**, the inability to hear out of one or both ears is a crushing blow. Many times, the diagnosis of this sudden-onset hearing loss and tinnitus includes the medical term 'idiopathic', which is the nice way of saying 'we have no idea why you woke up one day with this terrible hearing loss'. The most important advice for somebody who experiences a sudden change in hearing is to seek out the *immediate* assistance of a hearing healthcare specialist. It is possible, although not guaranteed, that immediate pharmaceutical intervention can recover some or all the hearing.

I HAVE BEEN WITH DR. WORTH SINCE SHE STARTED IN BUSI-
ness; fifteen years ago at least. I have always had individualized professional service that has met all of my hearing needs. I had a sudden
hearing loss and Cathy Worth treated me with compassion and understanding in what was a very traumatic situation. Cathy was a tremendous help to me. I have recommended Cathy Worth to many of my
friends and they all have been satisfied.

Patty B.
Patient at Capitol Hearing, New Mexico
Excellence In Audiology Member

MY TINNITUS WAS GETTING LOUDER AND MORE PERSISTENT.
A&E not only got me hearing well, but I finally lost that ringing! My life
has improved by leaps and bounds.

Elizabeth V.
Patient at A&E Audiology, Pennsylvania
Excellence In Audiology Member

CHAPTER 9

SHOULDN'T MY TREATMENT BE GUARANTEED?

Healthcare is notorious for no guarantees. Nearly every one of us knows that medical care can go horribly wrong. Guarantees are controversial in all kinds of healthcare including audiology. Many of my colleagues are upset by the very idea of the word **guarantee**. One even huffed-and-puffed at me saying, "what do you think you're doing with this guarantee nonsense? We are not operating a car shop, installing mufflers, and guaranteeing them for five thousand miles. We are doctors, dammit." (Feel free to conjure up an image of some stuffy doctor banging his fists on the table—that is close to what actually happened!)

His doctor ego was mightily offended. But I doubt you will be, with the challenge of deciding who should be your family's *trusted* hearing healthcare specialist. So, yes, I think there should be a guarantee! In fact, many guarantees!

1. **If you are not satisfied with your treatment or patient experience, *our team of specialists will make it right, guaranteed.***

2. **Also, the quality of the hearing and tinnitus treatment itself is *guaranteed for life*.**

If ever the proper treatment originally achieved somehow begins to fail, we will welcome you back and do everything we can to correct the problem and get you hearing your absolute best. With that said, we cannot ignore the progression of the disorder and must account for these changes in your auditory system and adjust prognosis accordingly.

3. **You also have a safety in numbers guarantee.**

The diagnostic and prescriptive methods and state-of-the-art technology we use have been used by top hearing healthcare specialists nationwide to treat more than one million patients successfully.

4. **You also have my guarantee that *every* hearing healthcare specialist and treatment specialist at my offices have been not only academically educated but also *thoroughly* trained.**

They all follow the same proven method to diagnose needs, plan the best and personalized treatments for every patient, and manage for best results from day one through after care. There is nobody "learning on the job" at my practices—ever! All patient care is supervised and reviewed. We also invest in frequent state-of-art clinical continuing education for our team exceeding all state licensing requirements. Above and beyond.

5.   You also have *my guarantee of exceptional courtesy and customer service.*

Yes, you are my patient, but we can be honest about this— my practice is not just a healthcare provider, it is a business. As such, it has, in my opinion, a responsibility to you, as the patient, to always tell the whole truth and nothing but the truth, prescribing in the patient's best interest and delivering the best possible treatment and outcomes.

There is also a second, separate set of responsibilities to you as a customer, including access, convenience, responsiveness, and "red carpet service."
We include these five guarantees in your treatment program.

So, let's start here: ***I can guarantee you the best, most thorough audiology exam and treatment plan at your local Excellence In Audiology™ member-clinic, and I encourage you to come in for it now!***

THIS OFFICE IS AMAZING! FROM THE OFFICE STAFF TO THE AU-
diologists, everyone is professional and courteous. I've had questions and concerns and I'm able to get answers by phone or a quick appointment to stop in. Would highly recommend to anyone who is looking for an audiologist. Easy payment plan that includes check ins, batteries, and anything else I need to hear my very best!

Sherrie M.
Patient at Intermountain Audiology, Utah (St. George)
Excellence In Audiology Member

PREVENTING DECLINE

CHAPTER 10

How to Get More Information

There are several ways to get information about a hearing healthcare practice. First, I want to address the ways I do not recommend.

I do not recommend Yelp. Yelp is, unfortunately, not at all what it seems and is frequently the subject of lawsuits from business owners and under regulatory scrutiny centered around the poorly policed manipulation of reviews and even flooding of fake reviews by "bots" no less! Some companies can use Yelp as competitive warfare while other companies turn around and sell the business owner under negative-review-assault "reputation management services." So, beware! Get the information you need from truly trusted sources.

Google is a great starting point and a valuable place to check out patient reviews and rankings. It takes effort to put together ones' thoughts and go online and leave a review. Before starting treatment, always check out the quantity and quality of reviews for hearing healthcare practices in your community.

First, the best thing to do is make certain you get all your questions answered by the hearing healthcare specialist and the practice's treatment coordinator. Do not hold back. Put them on the spot. Be assertive. Do not feel you have to be deferential to the guy in the white coat (which is part of the reason I do not wear a white coat, ever!). My own goal in this is to have every patient and every family member fully knowledgeable about every aspect of the treatment so that they have **zero** anxiety.

Second, visit ***ExcellenceInAudiology.org***. This is, as its name states, an organization of carefully chosen hearing healthcare practices and providers that have joined together to provide carefully curated, vetted, authoritative, accurate, and understandable patient and family information. This can definitely help you decide based on the questions you want answers to.

Finally, if you have a quick follow-up visit scheduled, these are wonderful opportunities to either ask questions you may have missed the first time or get further details from your provider directly. You will always leave our office with our treatment coordinator's name, email, and phone number.

Now that you know where to get your most burning audiology questions answered, here are some simple tips I have amassed over the years to help you easily and effectively get the information you need:

How to Get Your Questions Answered

- **Make a list.** The easiest way to get what you want is to know it in advance. Make a list of the various questions you have when they arise so you can quickly and easily go down the list to assure you have got the right answers for the right questions.

- **Bring it with you.** Take the list with you when you go for your audiology visit. That way you have the questions at hand, at the right place, at the right time. If you are calling in to get answers, you can also have the list ready and tick off one question for every answer you receive.

- **Record the answers.** If your hearing healthcare specialist, or their receptionist, speaks too fast or you cannot keep up while writing the answers down, why not record them (or at least ask them to slow down!)? Your cell phone likely has a "record" feature and, if not, there are many affordable micro-recorders on the market today.

- **Double check.** Finally, make sure you have the right answer by double checking with your practitioner or their receptionist or assistant.

Knowing where to find the information you need is only half the battle; follow these tips and you will know how to get what you are looking for as well.

Regardless of how many questions you have, or your comfort level with technology, phone calls or in-person visits, your hearing healthcare specialist should offer an option that fits your schedule and makes all your unresolved issues crystal clear.

I WENT INTO THIS HEARING APPOINTMENT NOT REALLY EX-
pecting anything. I walked out with head held high, having received great service from Kyle (Dr. Woods) and all the staff. The doctor was awesome, very informative and kind.

I was brought to tears when I heard clearly for the first time! I want to thank you, Kyle, for giving me back my hearing—I appreciate you and the staff at your office, and everything you did for me.

God bless you and your family.

Guy N.
Patient at Modern Hearing Solutions, Ohio
Excellence In Audiology Member

EXCELLENT EXPERIENCE! UNDERSTOOD MY HUSBAND'S PROB-
lems immediately and remedied the situation within 24 hours . . . not days or weeks! Gentle and understanding. Highly recommended!! This 'young at heart' man loves what he's doing! Our world needs more kind, honest and truly genuine people like John Nobile! Thank you!

Mary P.
Patient at Nobile Hearing Aid Center, Florida
Excellence In Audiology Member

CHAPTER 11

How to Pay for The Medical Treatment of Hearing Loss and Tinnitus

Assuming you are new to this, or perhaps you are one of the millions living with undertreated hearing loss, I hope by now that I have unequivocally answered the question of *'is it really necessary'* with a resounding YES!

While I hope you have learned a lot thus far in the book, I know many of you will still have your preconceptions and personal experiences with hearing loss that may weigh on your mind. Like me, maybe you had a grandparent (like my Gramma Mary) who walked around with beige bananas sticking out of their ears that whistled every time you gave them a hug. Perhaps you know somebody who got bamboozled into buying traditional hearing aids and now they use them as a paper weight. Or maybe you know somebody who was sold something from a door-to-door hearing aid widget-pusher and now the salesman's phone is disconnected. Or maybe your parent thought the widget they found online would really help them hear better!

While these stories break my heart, I know they are true, and I know they cannot be ignored. These experiences are real, and they deserve to be acknowledged, and they must be talked about. As I mentioned earlier, there are 'bad apples' in every industry, even healthcare. But that does not mean we can throw out the baby with the bathwater.

The inspirational stories of the tens of thousands of people we positively affect cannot be silenced by the disenfranchised. The treatment of hearing loss and tinnitus offers 5 simple and straightforward medical benefits.

BENEFITS OF THE MEDICAL TREATMENT OF HEARING LOSS AND TINNITUS

1. **Increase in Quality of Life.** Just ask the over 2000 patients who have left us 5-Star reviews online about how we have positively affected their lives and the lives of their family members. You can also visit IMATestimonials.com to see our video testimonials and watch many of our patients tell their stories.

2. **Increase in Mental Sharpness (aka 'less senior moments').** Although it may be a stretch to say that people who treat their hearing loss are smarter than the rest of us (although I have heard patients tell their spouse '*well, now I am smarter than you!*'), research has shown us that individuals who treat their hearing loss have increased memory, increased attention, and increased processing speed.

3. **Reduced Experience of Tinnitus.** Nearly 70-80% of patients who undergo treatment note a significant decrease in experiencing tinnitus.

4. **Decreased Risk of Dementia.** The early treatment of hearing loss is the *most* modifiable risk factor for reducing the chances of developing dementia.

5. **Decreased Risk of Falling.** Falls in older adults is the #1 cause of injury-related deaths, the #1 cause of hospitalizations and the #1 cause of losing independence and having to leave your home.

Now that you understand the implicit value in treating your hearing loss and tinnitus... lets tackle the ugly matter of money.

I say "ugly" because nobody really likes talking about this. I have observed audiology students and seasoned hearing specialists stumble through the 'money conversation'. When there is a financial obstacle to treatment, most people are reluctant to admit it, offer other excuses; and, in turn, they cannot be helped by their treatment provider.

We must trust each other. When we have this discussion, it is entirely confidential—consider it happening in a "safe zone". Believe me, hearing healthcare providers get it—we have mortgages, kids, cars, college tuitions (both our own and our kids!), and we have family budgets that we must work within.

We never make a treatment decision a financial decision.

WHAT IS A REASONABLE FEE AND COST?

A comprehensive cognitive treatment program, including your visits, your treatment technology, etc., can cost anywhere from $175 per month to $237 per month. Most fall in between. Nearly 95% of my patients pay $214 per month for their treatment program. When adjusted for inflation, these prices are actually *way less* than what they were even a decade ago—despite the fact that technology and treatment outcomes have increased by leaps and bounds.

In addition, when you consider the costs of **not** treating hearing loss, these treatment plans are a steal! For example, depression in older adults is often attributed to untreated or *under*treated hearing loss and costs on average $8,000 every few years. The average amount of money spent on caring for a loved one hospitalized by a fall, including home renovation or moving, is $30,000 per incident. And when it comes to dementia, the average cost of caring for a loved one is $57,000 per year. Thus, treating hearing loss is a bona fide BARGAIN!

For your investment, you will be getting the carefully selected treatment plan that directly targets your hearing loss, tinnitus, and cognitive needs. Your prescription is an exact science and matched exactly to you, and only you. Your investment also includes the expertise of a specialist who is considerate, compassionate, and empathetic from beginning to end. Your investment includes everything you need; seriously, everything.

> *"The bitterness of poor quality remains long after the sweetness of low price is forgotten."*
>
> —BENJAMIN FRANKLIN

Gone are the days of patients having to pay large sums of money all up front. You should no longer be asked to fork over thousands of dollars up front. In fact, if you are told by any hearing healthcare specialist that you must pay the full $4,000-$10,000 up front for treatment—*please politely excuse yourself and find a new provider!*

WHAT IS A MEMBERSHIP PLAN?

Our core value is simple: **Treat Every Patient**. But, because money does not grow on trees and people do not like parting with large sums of hard-earned money (nor should they!), we had to come up with a way to increase access and affordability *for all!* I am proud to offer a treatment membership to all of my patients in all of my practices as it truly puts the **PATIENT FIRST**. The different plans allow me to help every patient, regardless of hearing loss, insurance benefit, financial need, or **credit score**. Yes, you read that right—if your credit is compromised for any reason, even if you have NO CREDIT, you will always be offered an affordable treatment program.

The three facts of 'hearing care' are:

1. **Hearing loss is a progressive degenerative disorder that will require long-term adaptative treatment.**

2. **Technology used to treat hearing loss is constantly improving.**

3. **The costs continue to increase.**

Membership programs protect each patient by ensuring that their hearing loss, tinnitus, and cognitive needs are always treated with the best available technology and services—and we offer these programs with *locked-in* pricing!

How to Offset Treatment Costs

Use of membership programs is customized to meet each patient's needs. One way that many patients cover the low monthly cost is by using their Flexible Spending Account (FSA), using their tax returns, and even 'writing off' the cost of treatment as a medical expense benefit on their tax returns (warning— this is not considered 'tax advice' and I do not play an accountant on TV; so always ask your financial specialist how to best proceed with all tax matters).

Membership Plans and Your Flex-Spending Account (FSA)

Flexible spending accounts are accessible through your employer benefit package that allows you to set aside a certain amount of money per year, TAX-FREE, to be used towards medical expenses. The medical treatment of hearing loss and tinnitus *is* a medical expense. Perhaps you already follow the "5 Ps to Success," (Proper Planning Prevents Poor Performance!) but in case you don't, this is one thing you want to plan early for so you can maximize the benefit. Many employees set higher limits than you think on the amount of flexible spending dollars you can contribute and access.

I have seen employees with as much as $2,500 and some with even $5,000 in flex-spending dollars available to them. Failure to sign up early could cost you more in out-of-pocket medical expenses, especially if your plan is not up and ready before you or a loved one needs to treat his or her hearing loss and tinnitus. If you have a new plan, work with your human resource contact to sign up early for next year in order to maximize your savings.

Membership Plans and Insurance Benefits

While many patients in America do not have 'the medical treatment of hearing loss and tinnitus' as a covered benefit (please don't shoot the messenger) some people do. As an example, there are several states that have a mandated benefit for state employees; there are even certain federal employees (i.e., postal workers) that have a set benefit that can be used once every certain number of years. One thing for sure is that an insurance plan that will cover the **total** cost of treatment is like 'winning the lottery' and is an exceedingly rare find.

Ultimately, even with insurance, the patient will most often still have some monthly out-of-pocket costs. Attempting to determine which health insurance programs do and do not offer a benefit is an insurmountable task, especially considering the constant changes to health insurance programs.

For those few who do have insurance benefits that will contribute to the cost of treatment and hearing technology, the good news is that you can combine your benefit with a membership plan to reduce your low fixed monthly payment even further. If your local Excellence In Audiology™ member-clinic accepts the benefit provided by your insurance plan, they can easily integrate the benefit; thus, adjusting your membership plan to an even lower monthly cost.

WHAT IF YOU STILL REALLY, REALLY CANNOT AFFORD TREATMENT?

As I said earlier, a core value at our practices is to *treat every patient*. And if I say it—I mean it. The only way to make this core value a reality is to offer treatment options to those who really, really cannot afford it. I am talking about the 5-10% of patients who do not have Medicaid coverage, the patients who will have less food for their family if they treat their hearing loss, and those who risk losing their home if they invest in treating their hearing loss. If this is you—do not worry, we can help you too. Our non-profit organizations offer treatment to those less fortunate and those with true needs. Speak to your Excellence In Audiology™ member-clinic to learn more about their program and how to easily qualify.

THIS PLACE HAS GIVEN LIFE BACK TO MY HUSBAND. HE HAS had Tinnitus for many years and never knew he could have so much relief. Thanks for changing our lives.

Jennifer R.
Patient at Arizona Balance and Hearing Aids, Arizona
Excellence In Audiology Member

I HAD ANOTHER WONDERFUL 4-MONTH CHECK UP WITH MY caring audiologist, Dr. Turri. Investing in good hearing with a clinician who is so knowledgeable & dedicated to helping me have the best hearing and balance I can have during my golden years is the best investment I could ever have made! Thank you, Dr. Turri!

Catherine D.
Patient at The Villages Health Audiology, Florida
Excellence In Audiology Member

PREVENTING DECLINE

CHAPTER 12

WHAT ARE THE TREATMENT OPTIONS?

If you or a loved one are ready for hearing healthcare, one of the first discussions to have with your specialist is *which treatment is right for you*; there might be more options than you had ever imagined.

Remember, this is not 1982 or 1992. It is not 2002 or even 2012. I should know, I have been to the world's second largest hearing aid museum (*now that I think about it—I never did ask 'where is the world's largest museum?'*). Today's technology isn't anything like it used to be—even if you or a loved one first started treating hearing loss only 5 years ago—things have changed significantly. Today's hearing healthcare is far more advanced, more sophisticated, and more patient-centered than any prior generation has experienced. If you or a family member had traditional hearing aids, it was medieval torture. Thankfully, the dungeon is gone too, replaced by ultra-modern patient comfort friendly offices.

If you are like most people, you associate the hearing office with traditional hearing aids, but times change and so too does the medical treatment of hearing loss and tinnitus. Since we hear with our brains, not our ears, it is important that the technology you use to treat your hearing loss is designed to address the cognitive needs of hearing loss. Traditional hearing aids make sounds louder—all sounds—which is annoying and gets in the way of hearing what others have to say. New technology, sometimes referred to as NeuroTechnology™, help you hear more naturally, in all listening environments, including noisy restaurants.

Using traditional hearing aids to treat hearing loss is like using a hammer to juice an orange (that was the most ridiculous analogy I could come up with, so I hope it gets my point across!). When it comes to treating hearing loss, there are many factors to consider including stage of hearing loss, experience of tinnitus, impact of hearing loss on memory and cognitive function, etc. Thus, using a device to treat hearing loss that is solely designed to amplify all sounds is rather ridiculous and limiting.

Today's treatment options come with near limitless choices to customize and be prescribed specific to a patient's hearing loss symptoms and cognitive needs. As an example, new technology can seamlessly perform in different listening environments by adapting stimulation patterns to suit the person's needs. New technology also offers the benefits of truly being hands-free. I often liken new technology to the infomercial adage *'set it and forget it'*. You can listen to your phone through new technology, you can listen to the TV through the new technology (no more arguing over the TV volume!), it can alert family members when you fall, it can even be programmed to turn on your coffee maker every morning (*I have to admit—I have never actually tried to set this up for fear of being yelled at by a patient if their coffee is too bitter and it's somehow my fault!*).

People who live with normal hearing never really have to think about their hearing. Hearing is a natural process that requires little, if any, effort. People with hearing loss deserve the same—and we can now offer each patient the ease of 'normal' hearing.

Oh, and did I mention—all of our treatment technology is invisible! I have always believed that our first priority is to meet the hearing, tinnitus, and cognitive needs of each patient. I also accept that many patients' first priority is vanity. Now we can easily achieve both!

I WAS IMPRESSED WITH CHRIS'S KNOWLEDGE, PROFESSION- alism, and care. I have a unique situation with my ears and had been told years ago my hearing loss and tinnitus could not be helped. Fortunately, that's not the case anymore thanks to Chris Sumer and his team! I appreciated the time Chris took with me. He took the time to review my records and he has changed my life.

Patti M.
Patient at Coastal Hearing Aids, California
Excellence In Audiology Member

CHAPTER 13

How to Know If You Are Under-Treating Your Hearing Loss

No medical treatment last forever.

Forty-two million people live with untreated hearing loss. And *millions* more live with **undertreated hearing loss!**

For starters, you might be wondering '*what is an undertreated medical disorder and how does it apply to hearing loss?*' An *under*-treated medical condition indicates that insufficient treatment, or inadequate treatment, is being applied to a medical condition. In hearing healthcare, *under*treated hearing loss lacks the necessary acoustic stimulation for improving one's cognitive function, reducing tinnitus, increasing a person's quality of life, increasing sound awareness (i.e. reducing the risk of falling) and reducing their risk of dementia. *Traditional hearing aids undertreat hearing loss.*

So, what is the difference between traditional hearing aids and technology used to treat hearing loss today? Let's cover this answer with a bullet-point approach as the differences are black and white:

Traditional Hearing Aids:

- Amplify all noises.

- Make it difficult to hear in background noise.

- Do not address neurocognitive deficits.

- Do not support long-term tinnitus relief.

- Typically require up-front full payment.

New Cognitive Treatment Technology

- Provides direct bio-acoustic stimulation to the brain.

- Addresses neurocognitive needs including:

- Memory Recall

- Selective Attention

- Processing Speed

- Direct treatment support for patients with tinnitus.

- Reduced fall risk with increased auditory awareness (*some technology options can alert family members if you have fallen*).

- Cognitive stimulation patterns that can decrease dementia risk.

- ***Affordable for all with simple membership plans!***

If you are like me, and you also use the 'Compare' button when searching for items online, allow me to simplify these differences:

When compared to traditional hearing aids, new treatment technology yields a:

- 20% improvement in hearing others speak in quiet situations with very little background noise (i.e. 20% improvement in hearing the clarity of others' voices at home and when one-on-one)

- 40% improvement in the ability to hear and understand speech in the presence of background noise and other competing sounds in the environment (i.e. you can hear *so much* more in a restaurant)

- 18% decrease in experiencing annoying or loud noises that cause discomfort and interrupt the ability to hear in background noise

- 28% improvement in the ability to hear in rooms with poor acoustics (i.e. theatres, galleries, churches, etc.)

With our innovative approach to treating your progressive-degenerative disorder, we stand committed to **updating your treatment plan every 48 months** (or sooner if needed!). This revolutionary approach to treating hearing loss ensures that you receive the best, most up-to-date medical treatment available to provide maximum cognitive stimulation. As your hearing, tinnitus, and cognitive needs change, so too must your treatment program. Today's treatment programs are designed to meet the needs of the progressive-degenerative nature of the disorder, both today and tomorrow.

GREAT EXPERIENCE! AFTER THE FIRST TWO APPOINTMENTS trying to determine best course of action for beginning of hearing loss and several years of tinnitus, Dr. Laura Vinopal and her staff have been very professional, informative, helpful. They have also been very patient with all my questions and told me all of my available treatment options.

After different hearing tests were performed, questions answered and consultation with Dr. Laura, I decided to jump in. So far I am pleasantly surprised with, they are easy to work with in and out for nightly charging and so far seem to help with clarification. It's early in the process of getting acclimated to the new treatment but so far so good, I'm keeping a positive outlook and hearing things more clearly!

I highly recommend a visit if you are on the fence. My wife is very pleased I finally made an appointment and started getting educated about the importance of my hearing.

Brad T.
Patient at Professional Hearing Care, Wisconsin
Excellence In Audiology Member

CHAPTER 14

NOW THAT YOU STARTED TREATMENT, WHAT ELSE CAN YOU DO TO PREVENT DECLINE?

What starts with a commitment to the medical treatment of hearing loss and tinnitus leads to a promise to take best care of yourself by following a holistic and comprehensive treatment plan. Our simple motto that *hearing care is health care* means it is important that we think beyond the ears and assure you live your best, healthiest, life. We remain steadfastly committed to helping each patient understand how (in addition to treating their hearing loss) they can actively age, remain confident and stay fiercely independent.

Like treating all major medical conditions, the initial prescription (be it a pill to reduce your cholesterol, a round of radiation, an injection to control A1C levels, etc.) *must* be combined with a healthy lifestyle. The body has an incredible ability to provide relief and heal itself—but only when given the right resources.

Excellence In Audiology™ member-clinics commit to a holistic approach to treating sound, mind, and body. We not only help you hear your best, but we can also help you live your best life as you age and prevent decline. From the technology we use to help you hear your best every day and keep you mentally sharp, we can also help you to increase overall health by discussing diet, supplements, and exercise.

What you hear matters.

Your brain is always on. Your ears are always on too. This means your brain is constantly stimulated by the vast neural network from your ears. *Until it is not.* Then what happens?

There is a general belief that activities which stimulate the mind, i.e., hearing, can help to slow cognitive decline. Data tells us that treating hearing loss may even slow the progression of dementia.

What starts out as subtle cognitive changes that are seemingly associated with aging, goes on to affect an older adults' day-to-day function. As we age, there are certain expected cognitive declines that we will all experience. However, with increased risk of cognitive decline and dementia associated with hearing loss, it is important to know the differences of 'normal aging', MCI (mild cognitive impairment) and dementia.

Early stages of significant cognitive decline (first seen in MCI) include problems with memory, language, thinking, judgement, and visual perception. Fortunately, most people are still 'with it' enough to notice these issues and can seek early intervention. Family and close friends may also notice a change. But these changes often are not severe enough to significantly interfere with daily life.

COMMON SIGNS AND SYMPTOMS OF COGNITIVE DECLINE INCLUDE:

- Memory loss, such as forgetting names, places, or recent events.
- Problems with organizing or planning — struggling with multi-tasking.
- Difficulty with recognizing faces.
- Difficulty finding words — often losing vocabulary.
- Misplacing items.
- Problems calculating a tip or paying bills.
- Slower recall, which could either be visual or verbal.

MCI along with hearing loss can increase your risk of later developing dementia caused by Alzheimer's or other neurological conditions. Which is why addressing risk factors early, such as the medical treatment of hearing loss (and others listed in Chapter 6), is critical to preventing dementia.

The proper medical treatment of hearing loss and tinnitus is designed to provide the auditory feedback and cognitive stimulation your brain **needs**.

What you feed your body matters.

Much like an expensive car, your brain functions best when it gets only premium fuel. Eating high-quality foods that contain lots of vitamins, minerals, and antioxidants nourishes the brain and protects it from oxidative stress—the "waste" (free radicals) produced when the body uses oxygen—which can damage cells.

Diet

Unfortunately, just like an expensive car, your brain can be damaged if you ingest anything other than premium fuel. If substances from "low-premium" fuel (such as what you get from processed or refined foods) get to the brain, it has little ability to get rid of them. Diets high in refined sugars, for example, are harmful to the brain. In addition to worsening your body's regulation of insulin, they also promote inflammation and oxidative stress. Multiple studies have found a correlation between a diet high in refined sugars and impaired brain function.

Just as there is no magic pill to prevent cognitive decline, no single almighty brain food or supplement can ensure a sharp brain as you age. Nutritionists emphasize that the most important strategy is to follow a healthy dietary pattern that includes a lot of fruits, vegetables, legumes, and whole grains.

With that said, certain foods in this overall scheme are particularly rich in healthful components like omega-3 fatty acids, B vitamins, and antioxidants, which are known to support brain health and often referred to as 'brain foods'. Incorporating many of these foods into a healthy diet on a regular basis can improve the health of your brain, which could translate into better mental function.

Research shows that the best brain foods are the same ones that protect your heart and blood vessels, including the following:

- **Green, leafy vegetables.** Leafy greens such as kale, spinach, collards, and broccoli are rich in brain-healthy nutrients like vitamin K, lutein, folate, and beta carotene. Research suggests these plant-based foods may help slow cognitive decline.

- **Fatty fish.** Fatty fish are abundant sources of omega-3 fatty acids, healthy unsaturated fats that have been linked to lower blood levels of beta-amyloid—the protein that forms damaging clumps in the brains of people with Alzheimer's disease. Eating fish 1-2 times a week can be healthy for your brain (but be sure to choose varieties that are low in mercury, such as salmon, cod, canned light tuna, and pollack). If you are not a fan of fish, ask your doctor about taking an omega-3 supplement, or choose terrestrial omega-3 sources such as flaxseeds, avocados, and walnuts.

- **Berries.** Flavonoids, the natural plant pigments that give berries their brilliant hues, also help improve memory, research shows. In a 2012 study published in Annals of Neurology, researchers at Harvard's Brigham and Women's Hospital found that women who consumed two or more servings of strawberries and blueberries each week delayed memory decline by up to two-and-a-half years.

- **Tea and coffee.** The caffeine in your morning cup of coffee or tea might offer more than just a short-term boost! In a 2014 study published in The Journal of Nutrition, participants with higher caffeine consumption scored better on tests of mental function. Caffeine might also help solidify new memories, according to further research. Investigators at Johns Hopkins University asked participants to study a series of images and then take either a placebo or a 200-milligram caffeine tablet. More members of the caffeine group were able to correctly identify the images on the following day.

- **Walnuts.** Nuts are excellent sources of protein and healthy fats, and one type of nut in particular might also improve memory. A 2015 study from UCLA linked higher walnut consumption to improved cognitive test scores. Walnuts are high in a type of omega-3 fatty acid called alpha-linolenic acid (ALA), which helps lower blood pressure and protects arteries. That's good for both the heart and brain.

In considering that poor diet is now the leading killer globally and mental disorders account for the largest burden of global disability, the fact that diet appears to play a role in mental as well as physical health (as well as increasing the risk of dementia) must be taken very seriously.

Supplements

Yes, proper diet is critical. However, there are a variety of supplemental nutritional needs that are difficult to come by (even with a great diet) that our brains require as we age to help maintain sharp mental acuity and positive cognitive function. Natural supplements can combat certain health, lifestyle, and environmental factors that can increase the risk of cognitive decline and dementia, including:

- *Inflammation*
- *Poor Diet*
- *Insulin Resistance*
- *Lack of Exercise*
- *Poor Sleep*
- *High Blood Pressure*

5 FOODS FOUND TO IMPROVE BRAIN FUNCTION

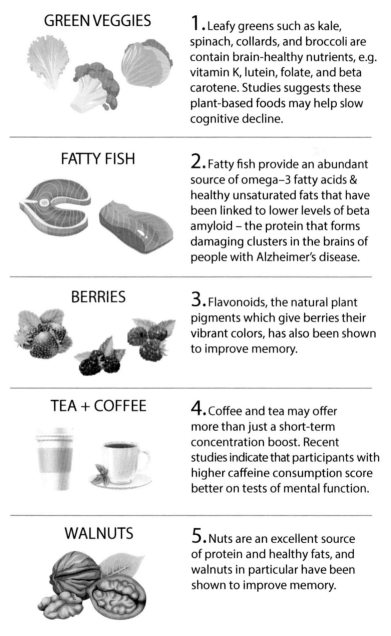

GREEN VEGGIES

1. Leafy greens such as kale, spinach, collards, and broccoli are contain brain-healthy nutrients, e.g. vitamin K, lutein, folate, and beta carotene. Studies suggests these plant-based foods may help slow cognitive decline.

FATTY FISH

2. Fatty fish provide an abundant source of omega–3 fatty acids & healthy unsaturated fats that have been linked to lower levels of beta amyloid – the protein that forms damaging clusters in the brains of people with Alzheimer's disease.

BERRIES

3. Flavonoids, the natural plant pigments which give berries their vibrant colors, has also been shown to improve memory.

TEA + COFFEE

4. Coffee and tea may offer more than just a short-term concentration boost. Recent studies indicate that participants with higher caffeine consumption score better on tests of mental function.

WALNUTS

5. Nuts are an excellent source of protein and healthy fats, and walnuts in particular have been shown to improve memory.

- *Toxins*
- *Stress*
- *Social Isolation*

Below is a short list of some of the most effective supplements available today that support healthy cognitive function as we age.

CoQ10 (Coenzyme Q10)

This naturally occurring antioxidant that reduces the proliferation of free radicals is produced in the human body for cellular growth and maintenance. Unfortunately, levels of CoQ10 decrease as we age. CoQ10 supports nerve health, the protection of brain tissue from oxidative damage and reduce the action of harmful compounds that can lead to brain disease. In addition, Coq10 supports healthy cardiovascular function and may reduce the risk for repeat heart attacks and helps combat side effects of cholesterol-lowering statins.

Ginkgo Biloba

This naturally occurring ingredient derived from a tree in Asia can support a healthy inflammation response, supports the production of important brain-building factors, supports recovery from heavy metal/mold exposure, supports healthy blood flow, and supports the brain's repair from physical trauma.

Phosphatidylserine

This hard to say but simple ingredient supports a healthy blood sugar response, provides important building factors, and supports the brain's recovery from trauma. The 80+ million Americans living with diabetes or pre-diabetes are at particular risk of cognitive decline given the inability of the body to effectively manage glucose levels.

Coffee Fruit Extract

Derived from the same plant as the coffee bean (although often discarded in favor of the coffee bean!) helps support healthy blood sugar response and increases the brain's production of key building factors like brain-derived neurotrophic factor (BDNF) that build proteins found in the brain.

Yamada Bee Propolis

Extracted by bees and combined with specific plant proteins to help protect themselves, this supplement support healthy inflammation response, supports healthy blood sugar levels, supports the production of brain-building factors, supports recovery from exposure to heavy metal and mold exposure, supports normal blood flow, and supports brain repair from trauma.

Turmeric

Many Americans have this tasty spice in their kitchen cabinets, but too often left un-used! Curcumin, a substance found in Turmeric helps support healthy inflammatory response, provides brain-building compounds, and supports recovery from heavy metal and mold exposure.

Gotu Kola

This herbal extract (from the parsley family) is commonly found in traditional Chinese medicine. This derivative has been used for thousands of years and helps support a healthy inflammatory response, healthy blood flow, and supports brain repair from trauma.

Don't forget, what you do with your body matters too!

Have you heard that '**sitting is the new smoking**'? When we sit around and let our brains wonder '*what will be the cause of our demise*', most of us think about heart disease, diabetes, cancer, dementia, old-age, pneumonia, disease, etc. But, according to new data (as recent as the day I wrote this chapter in 2021!) the chair you sit in most is one of the biggest threats to your health. No, this doesn't mean you should immediately go and throw out your favorite chair, rather, it's time to consider having '*the talk*' with your favorite chair and let it know you need to get out and stretch your legs more!

Rather than try and come up with my own novel scary statement about how we need to get up from our chairs and be more active, I believe Dr. James Levine, a professor of medicine at the Mayo Clinic has said it best:

> "*Sitting is more dangerous than smoking, kills more people than HIV, and is more treacherous than parachuting. We are sitting ourselves to death.... the chair is out to kill us.*"
> —Dr. James Levine, Mayo Clinic

To put it in to perspective—we were not designed to sit. Think about it—we are bi-pedal for a reason and sitting isn't the reason. The body is meant to stay in perpetual motion until rest is required. Humans have been on the planet way longer than the chair was invented.

If right about now you are thinking '*but I exercise, so this can't apply to me*', unfortunately that doesn't hold true. Yes, exercise

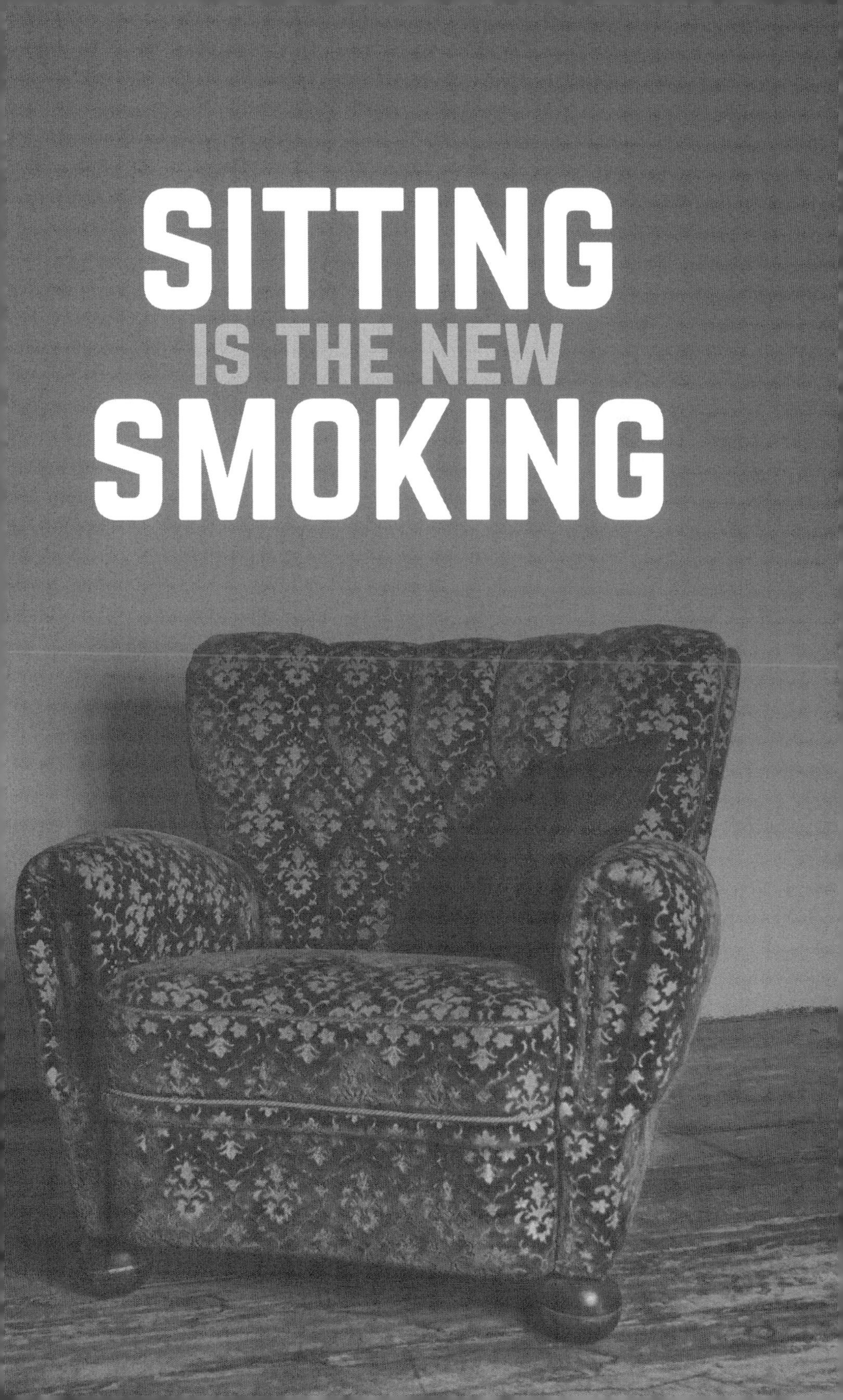
SITTING
IS THE NEW
SMOKING

is good for you, and we all need to do more of it; but it doesn't negate the damage we do to our bodies by sitting for extended periods of time, day after day. Thus, it stands to reason that more exercise is not the answer to sitting too much. Sadly, 10 hours of stillness in a chair (which is not uncommon for people at work) cannot be offset by 1 hour of exercise.

Sitting for long periods of time changes you. It changes your metabolism. It changes the way your body behaves and stores nutrients. In fact, your metabolism can slows down by as much as 90% after only 30 minutes of sitting. (If you are wondering—I too am guilty of owning a fancy machine-powered standing desk that allows me to stand while at work—but I do not use it nearly as much as I should!).

Sitting too long increases the risk of nearly everything that can kill you, including increased rates of:

- Type-2 Diabetes
- cardiovascular disease
- obesity
- disturbed sleep

And increased risk of:

- back and neck pain
- cancer
- deep vein thrombosis
- anxiety and depression
- Alzheimer's and dementia
- premature death

So, what is the best way to combat 'sitting too much'. While this is particularly hard for those who work at a desk, it can also be a challenge for many people living with the social isolation that accompanies hearing loss. For starters, get in the habit of standing and/or walking at least once every 20 minutes. With the advent of computers that fit on our wrist, we can now set up simple reminders that get us to 'stand'. I particularly like the smart-watches that will not stop reminding you until you actually stand up!

The goal is to gradually extend our periods of standing and increase the frequency of taking short walks. This is not about engaging in a newfound cross-fit exercise program, rather increase the frequency (not the intensity) of physical movement. There are many things we can do every day to increase our standing-to-sitting ratio. When you are at home or work, here are some simple things you can do each day to change your sitting habit:

- *drink a lot of water* (while good for you, this also has the advantage of making you walk to the bathroom more often),

- *talk and walk* (when reaching out to a friend or colleague on the phone, take the call 'to-go' and walk around),

- *pay your bills standing up* (my mother always sits at her desk to pay her bills- mother, please stand at the counter-height island and pay your bills!),

- *meet up for a coffee and a walk* (next time you meet somebody for a coffee why not walk and talk rather than sitting down),

- park further from the entrance to wherever you are

going (i.e., take the furthest available spot at the super-market), and

- *take the stairs* (now that you drink lots of water, try and use the bathroom furthest away in your house, prefera-bly up or downstairs!).

In addition to the extra movement you will have from sitting less, a little bit of exercise truly goes a long way. A simple reg-ular exercise regimen can increase your metabolism, help you keep cancer, diabetes, heart disease and obesity at bay, and keep you socially active (i.e., the opposite of social isolation!). While everybody has their preferred physical activity, my top two are swimming and pickleball. And if you do not know what pickle-ball is—it is the fastest growing sport in our country for those over 50 years young. Although I have unofficially nicknamed the game 'tiny tennis', it provides *BIG* benefits by increasing heart rate, burning calories, requiring hand-eye coordination, boost-ing your balance, and I guarantee you will smile when you play (which is a great workout for your face muscles!).

Always take the opportunity to talk to your hearing health-care provider and primary care physician about a holistic ap-proach to living your best life.

NOW THAT YOU STARTED TREATMENT, WHAT ELSE CAN YOU DO TO PREVENT DECLINE?

PREVENTING DECLINE

THE FOLKS AT CENTRAL MAINE AUDIOLOGY ARE WONDERFUL.
Through their expertise and caring they have significantly increased my quality of life. My hearing had become so poor that family members were irritated by my constant requests for repeating their words and I couldn't even hear the birds chirping at my feeders.

Now that has all changed. I am hearing things that were lost to me for years. Music is more enjoyable, my family is happier and the sounds of nature are once again present in my life.

Thakn you all at Central Maine Audiology, (especially Dr. Cropper, Abbey and the team) for your hard work and kind attention!

Steven W.
Patient at Central Maine Audiology, Maine
Excellence In Audiology Member

CHAPTER 15
LET'S CELEBRATE!

Having to treat your hearing loss and use technology to acti-vate the brain (*even though its invisible!*) is not something that most of us think about or plan for as we age—but now that you are here—lets embrace it and celebrate it!

From the moment you accept your hearing loss for what it is and get the treatment you need, and deserve, you are commit-ting to yourself and your family to live your best possible life, remain confident and fiercely independent.

Does treating hearing loss mean things in your life have to change? Yes—***FOR THE BETTER!!***

One of the first things I say to my patients when we begin treatment is '*Welcome Back*'. Welcome back to the world of the hearing and the world where you do not have to work so hard to be a part of the conversation. I have spent countless hours with patients talking about how their treatment has positively impacted their lives and the lives of their family members.

As we go through the treatment process, I often ask patients to reflect on what it was like living with untreated hearing loss and how it made them feel. Over the years I have made notes of what my patients say when referring to *what it used to be like when they had hearing loss.* Here are the most common feelings that patients have shared with me about their experience living with untreated or *under*treated hearing loss.

My hearing loss made me feel . . .

- *embarrassed.*
- *insecure.*
- *lonely.*
- *crazy.*
- *inadequate.*
- *old.*
- *foolish.*
- *afraid.*
- *forgotten.*
- *diminished.*
- *frustrated.*
- *demented.*
- *forgetful.*
- *out of balance.*
- *like I had crickets in my ear.*
- *like an argumentative spouse.*
- *like my life was over.*
- *like my life was not worth living.*

When you begin treating your hearing loss and tinnitus and embrace a holistic approach to active aging you are embarking on a journey. By treating your hearing loss, you are agreeing to invest in the process and to be patient. Treating hearing loss is an adaptive process that takes time. While most patients go from hearing good to great in under 30 days, some can take longer. In fact, for our patients with the most pressing tinnitus that interferes with daily life—the brain can take up to 18 months to adapt and suppress the neural-driven experience of tinnitus.

You will have to learn some new things, simple things, like charging your technology at night, remembering to clean the technology regularly and learning how to answer your cell phone so you can hear it more clearly through your new technology. Fortunately, I can report that after 20 years of being an audiologist, I've yet to meet a patient that was too old to learn something new (just in case you were thinking about backing out at this point!).

I promise, in fact I guarantee, that the time, financial investment and sacrifices you make to treat your hearing loss will pay off in exponential dividends. I have often said to colleagues, the medical treatment of hearing loss and tinnitus is probably the best bang for the buck any patient could ever get. There are so many ways you and your family can celebrate your new hearing; I often tell patients that perhaps the best way is to sit down over a nice meal and simply have a conversation—experience what it feels like to be part of the conversation, what it feels like to listen with minimal effort and what it feels like to know you have given yourself a chance at having the best possible life.

DR. ALISON HOFFMAN AND ADVANCED HEARING CENTER changed my life! I can't say enough good things about her and her staff. They are kind and understanding and most importantly great at what they do! I was having a lot of issues at home and at work due to my significant hearing loss but had put off getting treatment because of the cost. I was given different payment options that I could afford!

Don't wait like I did because your quality of life will instantly become so much better! I highly highly recommend you make an appointment with Dr. Hoffman and her team!

Mary C.
Patient at Advanced Hearing Center, New York
Excellence In Audiology Member

Aging is *inevitable.*
Decline is *optional.*

What do **you** choose?

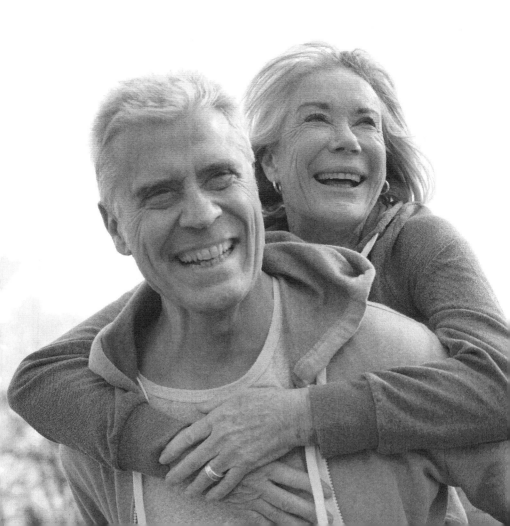

FAQS

Here is a handy-dandy resource section for you and your loved ones to help guide you through some of the most Frequently Asked Questions (FAQs).

Is it really such a big deal if I do not treat my hearing loss?

Unfortunately, yes. Untreated hearing loss is linked to life-threatening medical conditions including mental decline, dementia, falls, hospitalizations, and even pre-mature death. The time to act is now as hearing loss cannot be 'managed' by just making people speak louder!

Who are some familiar faces that have treated their hearing loss?

To name a few... Whoopi Goldberg, Stephen Colbert, President Ronald Reagan, William Shatner, Jody Foster, Halle Berry, Peter Townsend, President Bill Clinton, and Huey Lewis.

Will I be able to afford treatment?

Yes. Membership programs are more affordable than your cable and cell phone bills. Most patients can also take advantage of their insurance benefits and Health Savings Accounts to make their payments lower than the cost of coffee per day.

It is a great day when you can tell a patient that a treatment decision doesn't have to be a financial decision!

Is treating my hearing loss and tinnitus painful?

No. Modern treatment technology and testing procedures are painless. In fact, most of today's technology is completely invisible and so light weight.

How much work / family time will I miss because of treatment?

Not much, actually. After the initial visits, most appointments are anywhere from fifteen to forty-five minutes.

I am a snowbird and want to know what happens to me when I am not at home for several months per year?

If you are lucky enough to have that home-away-from-home, then we suggest you enjoy it to its fullest! We will provide you with all of the technology supplies and needs before you go away, and we are never more than a phone call away. If needed, we can even do a tele-health 'zoom conference call' and talk you through any troubles. We guarantee—treating your hearing loss will make your life better and never be a burden or stress.

What are some of the warning signs that I might have some signs of early-stage hearing loss?

The four most common signs of hearing loss are:

1. Difficulty following a conversation when there is background noise (i.e., at a restaurant).

2. Tinnitus (ringing/buzzing sounds in your ears and/or head).

3. Your family is telling you that you need help!

4. More 'senior moments' that you would like to admit!

What are some of the "side effects" of untreated tinnitus?

Tinnitus can have a profound impact on a person's ability to hear, concentrate, sleep and your emotional state of mind. Most often, tinnitus is caused by hearing loss and should be thought of as your *internal alarm* telling you that something is wrong and requires your attention asap!

What makes a hearing healthcare specialist (Audiologist or Board-Certified Hearing Instrument Specialist), more qualified than a PCP or an ENT?

Hearing healthcare providers specialize in the medical treatment of hearing loss and tinnitus. Whereas your PCP is your 'general health contractor' that oversees all your healthcare needs, and the ENT specializes in swallowing and speech, breathing and sleep issues, surgical intervention of hearing loss, allergies and sinuses, head and neck cancer, skin disorders, and facial plastic surgery.

Why should I choose a specialist to treat my hearing loss?

Unique treatment requirements and otherwise difficult auditory problems are common everyday scenarios for your hearing healthcare provider. In the interest of receiving the most efficient and effective treatment possible, choose a hearing healthcare specialist.

How do I know if my provider is an Audiologist or Hearing Instrument Specialist?

Only healthcare providers can belong to the Excellence In Audiology™ network of providers. Most Audiologist and Hearing Instrument Specialist are also accredited by the American Academy of Audiology (AAA), American Speech-Language-Hearing Association (ASHA) and/or the International Hearing Society (HIS).

What is a treatment coordinator?

During your initial consultation(s), you will usually be assigned a patient contact person—we call this person a "treatment coordinator"- with whom to schedule appointments, confer with scheduling and, of course, answer all questions you may have.

Why are follow-up visits important?

These are wonderful opportunities for your provider to 'fine-tune' your cognitive stimulation and maximize your treatment and for you to get further details or answer any lingering questions you may have.

Why is early treatment so important?

To put it simply: ***A Mild Hearing Loss is a Major Problem!*** Although we recommend that everybody over the age of 50 years young have regular hearing evaluations, you are never too young to treat your hearing loss at the first signs. Unfortunately, even a Stage 1 hearing loss (sometimes referred to as a 'mild hearing loss') can increase your risk of mental decline and dementia by as much as 200%! Like every medical condition, it is important to 'catch it early and treat it early!'.

Is there such a thing as a being 'too old' to start treatment?

No. Although many patients try to reason their way out of treatment by saying *'what's the point, I only have a few years to live'* the benefits of treatment, whether they be for 6 months or 6 years, positively impact your overall social, emotional, physical and cognitive health and may help you live longer!

What if I do not believe in treating my hearing loss (after all, my parents never did)?

Well, you're entitled to your opinion, but this is like saying you do not believe the earth is round (my apologies if I just offended any 'flat-earthers'). You can hide from it, pretend it is not there, refuse to acknowledge it or believe that you can 'manage' without medical intervention, but the simple fact remains—*if you are not aware of the potential risks, you are likely to suffer from them.*

What is tinnitus?

When the ear breaks down from age, noise exposure, medications, virus, genetics, etc., the nerves that travel from ear-to-brain break down. This results in a 'surge' of neural activity (referred to as *Central Gain*) that is perceived as sound. Nearly 90% of people with tinnitus have hearing loss (and vice versa).

Where should I start to look for treatment if I am concerned about my hearing loss (or for a loved one)?

If you suspect that you have hearing loss (or have been told by somebody to get your ears checked), go to the website **ExcellenceInAudiology.org** to find a local hearing healthcare provider that you can trust subscribes to best practices. Please, stay away from anybody who partakes in sleezy sales tactics.

Why should I address tinnitus?

Tinnitus is most often one of the first signs of hearing loss. Because hearing loss is gradual (for most patients) they often notice the ringing in their ears before noticing a change in hearing. This 'alarm' inside your head is telling you that something is wrong, and it needs to be medically addressed ASAP.

What is treatment technology?

The way we treat hearing loss today is different (aka *way better!*) then even a few years ago. While traditional hearing aids were good at making sounds louder—they made EVERY sound louder—even the ones that were harmful and annoying! Today's technology is specifically designed to address the cognitive aspects of hearing loss, tinnitus and associated cognitive deficiencies. When treatment is done right, you can hear as *naturally* as possible.

What are the primary benefits of treatment?

To summarize, the five medical benefits of treatment include:

- Increase in quality of life and relationships at home and with friends.
- Reduced experience of tinnitus.
- Decreased risk of falling (the #1 cause of injury-related death in older adults).
- Increased mental acuity.
- Reduced risk of mental decline and dementia.

How do I get started with treatment?

It is simple: just make an appointment with your local hearing healthcare provider (which you can find on the website *ExcellenceInAudiology.org*) for an initial consultation. Most practices will offer a free initial consultation to see if you are a good candidate for their treatment program.

How will treatment impact my brain?

New treatment technology has been found to effectively increase memory recall, processing speed and selective attention. The increased brain activity from treatment may also eliminate your increased risk of falling and losing your independence at home.

Is medical treatment of hearing loss and tinnitus appropriate if I am in my 30's or 40's?

Yes, especially because we now know that the early treatment of hearing loss is the #1 modifiable lifestyle factor to reduce your risk of developing cognitive decline and dementia.

Why are traditional hearing aids still sold?

Frankly, I have no idea! If it were up to me, I would ban the sale of all traditional hearing aids. I believe that as medical professionals we are ethically bound to only provide the best treatment available and never compromise on patient care.

Is so-called "invisible technology" effective?

Yes. As the technology we use to treat hearing loss continues to advance, the 'packaging' this technology comes in has become smaller and nearly invisible. While providing the *right* treatment is the first priority, we are able to make your technology as discrete and invisible as possible. Long gone are the 'beige bananas' on people's ears!

What are some of my payment options in addition to insurance?

Our core value is to *treat every patient*. In order to do this, we have met the challenge of making treatment affordable for all. Gone are the days of patients and families paying thousands of dollars up front (in fact, if you are ever told that you must pay in full—I suggest you politely excuse yourself from the appointment and run far, far away!). With membership programs that are compatible with insurance benefits and Health Savings Accounts (HSA's), we can help patients afford medical treatment for a few dollars per day.

What if I have a "hearing emergency" before or after office hours?

If you are experiencing a hearing emergency that cannot wait for regular office hours, most practices have a special number to call before, during or after business hours. If this information is not given to you readily, ask how your hearing healthcare practice handles office emergencies. We know that 'stuff happens' and that it doesn't always happen 9-5pm Monday through Friday, which is why we are always available to our patients.

Do I have to worry about moisture or sweat hurting my hearing technology?

While full submersion of any computerized technology is never encouraged, today's hearing technology is both moisture and dust resistant and can stand up to a beating!

Can I wear a mask while I wear my hearing technology?

A lot has changed in recent years and now that masks have become 'normal' in today's society, you need not worry that they interfere with treating your hearing loss. Because most patients feel that treating their hearing loss is a 'natural' process and something they don't actively think about, we remind patients to be careful when wearing anything on their ears that can accidentally cause your technology to fall off and get lost. (Most new technology has a 'GPS homing beacon' built into it and you can use your phone to find any lost technology!).

In addition to treating my hearing loss, what else can I do to keep my mind and body healthy?

Treating hearing loss is one of many things that older adults can do to look and feel their best. A proper diet with brain healthy foods and supplements is a vital component to maintaining mental acuity and sharpness as we age. Talk to your hearing healthcare provider about 'what else' can be done to actively age.

VISIT

DrKeithDarrow.com

for more information about treatment,
Dr. Darrow's podcast, and to keep up
with Dr. Darrow's push for active aging.

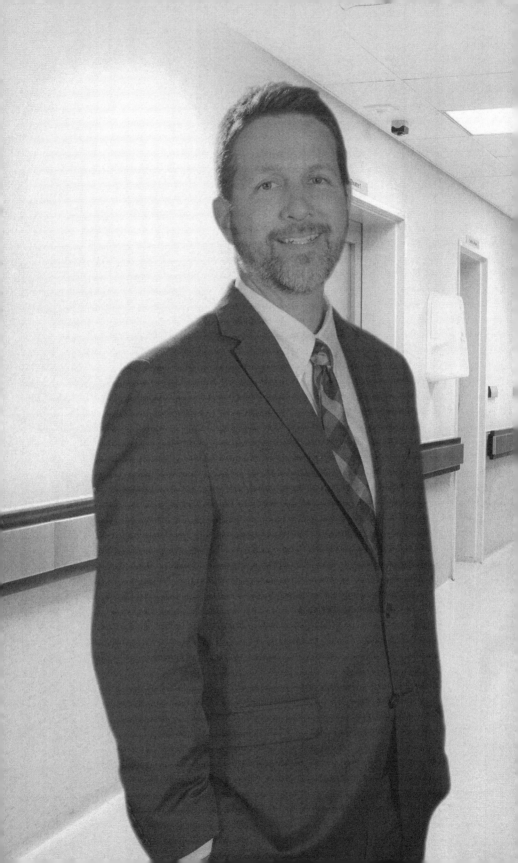

ABOUT THE AUTHOR

Dr. Darrow is a M.I.T. and Harvard Medical School trained Neuroscientist, Clinical Audiologist, Certified Dementia Prevention Educator, Certified Dementia Practitioner and Nationally Certified Alzheimer's Disease and Dementia Care Trainer. He is a former Clinical Professor at Northeastern University and is currently a tenured professor at Worcester State University. Dr. Darrow's clinical experience is vast and includes a clinical fellowship at the Department of Otolaryngology at Brigham and Women's Hospital, and he is co-founder of the Hearing & Brain Centers of America.

Dr. Darrow has chosen to lead the Excellence In Audiology™ movement across the country to improve the lives of the 42 million people living with untreated hearing loss. This expedition recruits the *best of the best* in hearing healthcare from across the United States and beyond to build a vast network of leading, life-changing, practitioners. This exclusive network brings together teams that share the same mission: *increase access, quality of service and exceed expectations for all of those suffering with hearing loss and tinnitus.*

His first Amazon.com best-selling book, *Stop Living In Isolation*, has been read by over one hundred thousand patients across the country and is heralded as the most informative resource in hearing healthcare. Dr. Darrow is a nationally recognized speaker, trainer, and researcher and has conducted research at the Massachusetts Eye and Ear Infirmary. His scientific findings and publications have been celebrated and cited over 950+ times.

THE NEXT STEP:

Your Customized Treatment Plan

When you are ready, or your loved one agrees that they need to take the next step, I urge you to schedule your customized treatment plan analysis and complimentary consultation. There is never a cost or an obligation to treatment in these appointments as we welcome the opportunity to educate you and your family members.

We encourage you to find an *ExcellenceInAudiology.org* center near you and always work with somebody you trust. While credentials and experience are important, you must feel that you are in the best hands and that your treatment will never be compromised.